D1199625

# SAVORY SWEET LIFE

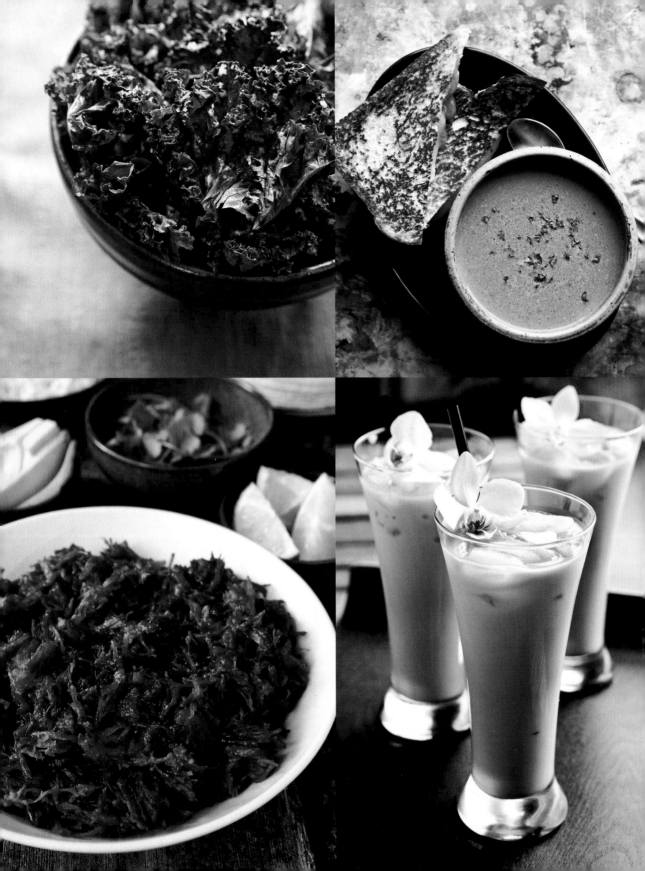

# SAVORY SWEET LIFE

## 100 Simply Delicious Recipes for Every Family Occasion

### ALICE CURRAH

WILLIAM MORROW
*An Imprint of HarperCollinsPublishers*

SOMERSET CO. LIBRARY
BRIDGEWATER, N.J. 08807

All photographs by Alice Currah except for page xi, by Arnold Gatilao.

SAVORY SWEET LIFE. Copyright © 2012 by Alice Currah. All rights reserved. Printed in the United States of America. No part of this book may be used or reproduced in any manner whatsoever without written permission except in the case of brief quotations embodied in critical articles and reviews. For information address HarperCollins Publishers, 10 East 53rd Street, New York, NY 10022.

HarperCollins books may be purchased for educational, business, or sales promotional use. For information please write: Special Markets Department, HarperCollins Publishers, 10 East 53rd Street, New York, NY 10022.

FIRST EDITION

Designed by Kris Tobiassen

Library of Congress Cataloging-in-Publication Data has been applied for.

ISBN 978-0-06-206405-9

12  13  14  15  16  ID / RRD  10  9  8  7  6  5  4  3  2  1

*For Rob, Abbi, Mimi, and Eli.*

Love you more (times infinity plus one).

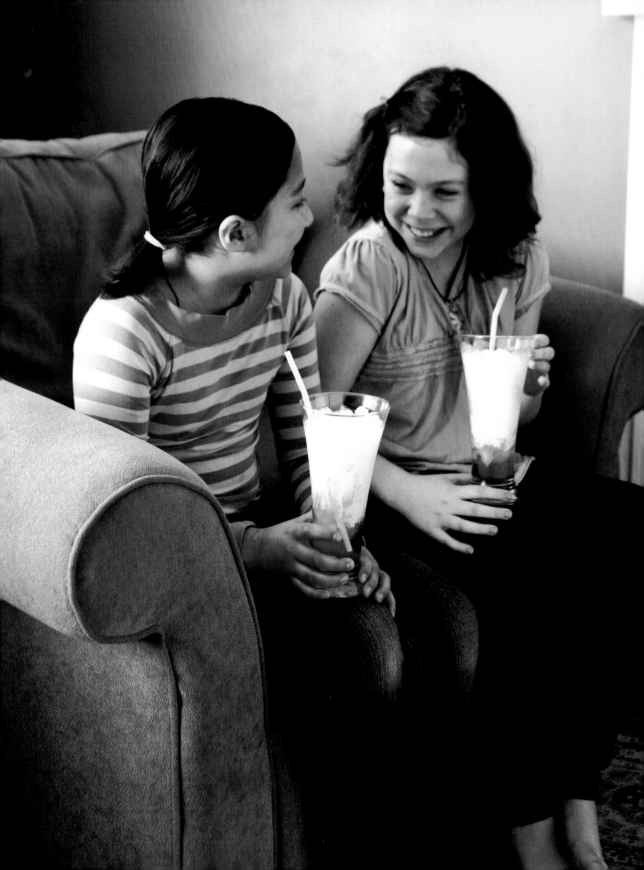

I don't like gourmet cooking or "this" cooking or "that" cooking. I like good cooking.

—JAMES BEARD

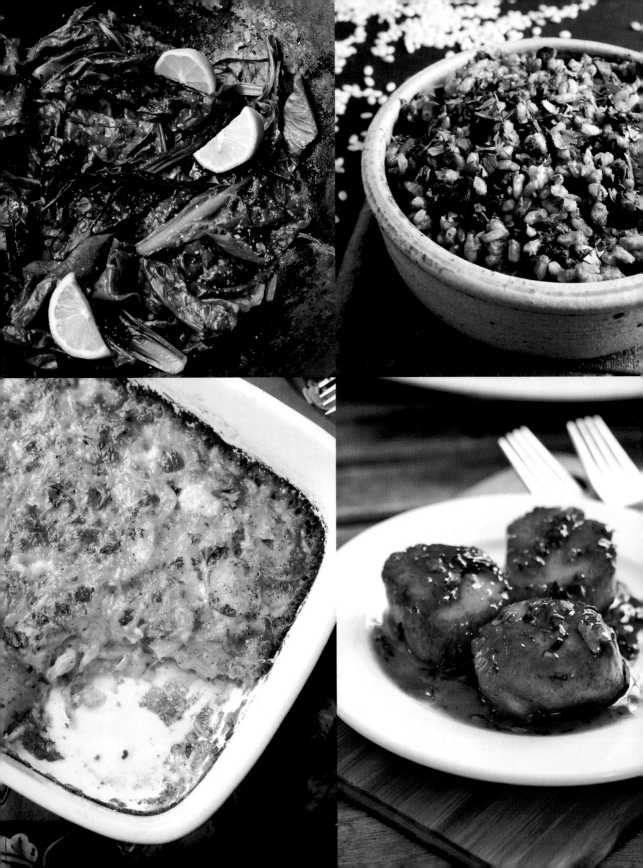

# CONTENTS

# FOREWORD

**BY REE DRUMMOND, THE PIONEER WOMAN**

*Alice and I met* for the first time at a conference in San Francisco. She introduced herself, then presented me with a small jar of sea salt from Puget Sound. We stood there and talked, and within a minute or two I knew a friendship had begun. Alice didn't bother with small talk or uncomfortable, introductory how-do-you-do's; instead she launched right into emotional, meaningful conversation as if those few minutes would be the only time we'd ever get to spend together. I remember our conversation as if it were yesterday.

When I returned home from the conference, I whipped up a batch of chocolate truffles . . . and sprinkled some of my Puget Sound sea salt over the top of each one. I stood back and admired the truffles, reflecting on what a unique, memorable gift the sea salt had been and what a sweet soul I'd met in Alice. In the years since, I've protected the little jar of salt as a precious treasure, using it only when I feel that what I'm cooking or baking is worthy of such a fine adornment. And whether it's dusting the top of salted caramels or buttered rosemary rolls, I always think of Alice when I use it.

I savor that sea salt, in much the same way Alice savors life.

Alice's contemplative appreciation for everyday joys is evident in her writing, whether on her website, Savory Sweet Life, or in her e-mail correspondence with me. Whatever the topic, she always manages to write something that makes me slow down, take a moment, and take her words to heart. In this time of hurried, hectic schedules and overflowing in-boxes, seeing a message from Alice always makes me smile because I know

I'm in for some sort of treat: a word of encouragement, a beautiful photo, or just a chuckle. Alice's silly sense of humor is the icing on the cake.

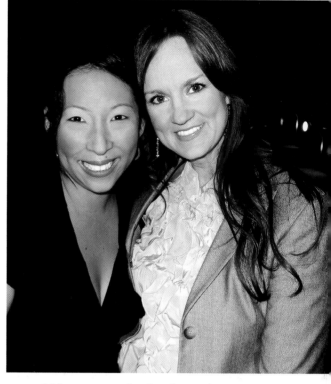

And then there's her food. I've been a fan of Alice's cooking blog from the beginning, mostly because she pours her heart and creativity into the things she cooks and bakes. Her ability to nail simple-but-delicious food is what keeps me coming back. I could marry her Caramelized Onion Clam Dip and live happily ever after with her Rustic Spiced Plum Tart. My kids, on the other hand, would eat her Caramel Corn every day for the rest of their lives and never tire of it. Yum!

I cheered for joy when I learned that Alice would be writing this book. And as I read it and inhaled not just the delicious recipes, but also her stories about how the food colors all the occasions and celebrations in her family, I settled in and savored every word. And my heart . . . well, it just felt happy.

I know the same thing will happen to you.

Love,
Ree

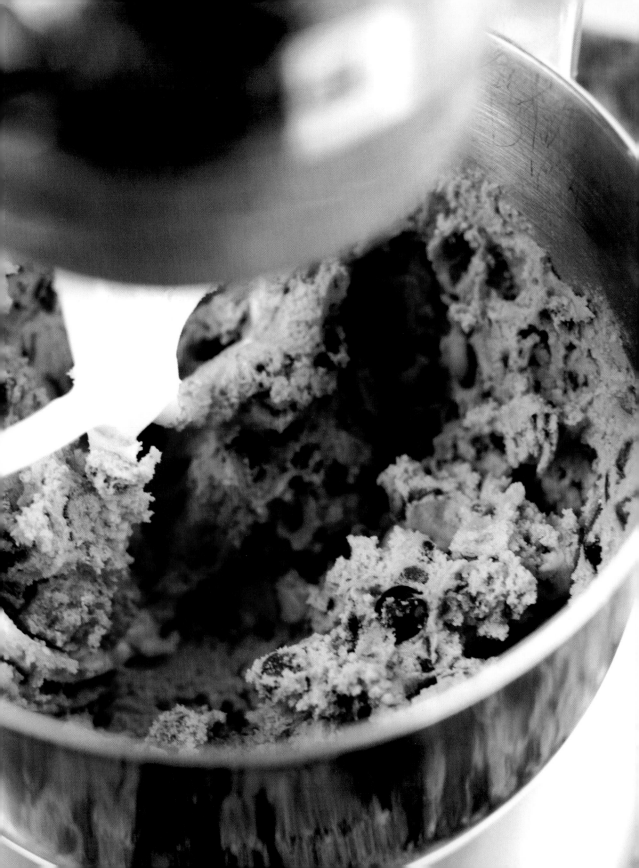

# INTRODUCTION

*When I close my eyes,* I can still remember vivid details about the dishes my mother prepared for my siblings and me when we were kids—dishes like spaghetti with sauce from a Prego jar, which was hardly difficult to make but comforting nonetheless because of the personal touches Mom added to make the recipe her own.

Most of Mom's meals were of the one-pot variety because both my parents typically worked twelve- to fourteen-hour days. Mom would make dinner in the morning before leaving for work so it would be ready for us when we came home from school hungry. In hindsight, we should have appreciated her spaghetti more.

I knew my father as a gardener long before it was considered cool to grow your own organic food. I grew up with four sisters and a brother in North Seattle, where Dad's garden was nearly as big in square footage as our tiny brick home. He grew all sorts of vegetables—red-leaf lettuce, spinach, broccoli, cucumbers, squash, potatoes—and the chain-link fence around our property also served as an arbor for grapevines. We had an apple tree that produced small greenish-red apples, which we'd pick for Mom's homemade applesauce during the autumn months. I was convinced the apples from our tree were exotic because Mom's applesauce was the best. The only ingredients she ever added were a touch of cinnamon and a smidge of water.

My mother was a great cook, although she said her approach to cooking was too simple to be considered "good" home cooking. But I disagree. Her food was honest, comforting, and delicious. There were never leftovers and we always had enough. Cooking was her strength, but baking was another story. I don't recall her ever baking a single thing in our oven.

Fortunately for our family, we were blessed to have a wonderful elderly neighbor named Alice, after whom I was named. While she never married or had children of her own, we considered her our second grandmother, which she loved. She was short in stature but full of energy and stories of her travels to Africa and other exotic places. I loved her stories, but what I loved even more was her passion for baking.

Every Sunday we waited anxiously for our old olive-green rotary phone to ring. When Mom picked up the phone we would watch intently for signs that it was Alice inviting us to come visit her. Her enthusiastic voice was the only prompt we needed to know it was time to go. My sisters and I would get our shoes on as fast as we could and race to her house, fighting over who would ring the doorbell. When Alice opened her door, the aroma of freshly baked goods was always right behind her: apple pie, blueberry muffins, and a host of other treats.

Alice's baking had a way of making us feel loved and fortunate. Whether it was homemade cream puffs filled with vanilla-scented whipped cream, a fresh fruit pie with berries picked from her yard, or a batch of sugar cookies just out of the oven, everything she baked was scrumptious and every Sunday with Alice was special.

Every year Alice would bake each of us a beautifully decorated birthday cake. There was always a card attached with a one-dollar bill inside. We waited on pins and needles to see what our cake would look like. As soon as Alice called to let us know it was ready, we ran to her house and carefully carried home her masterpiece. Mom would insist we wait until after dinner to eat our cake, which was torture. When it was finally time for cake, Mom would cut eight small slices, with us stuffing our mouths as quickly as we could, hoping for a shot at a second piece. Our family never celebrated birthdays with presents—being together and Alice's special birthday cakes were the only gifts I ever needed.

My family has always believed that I supernaturally inherited Alice's baking genes, and I'll be forever grateful to her for the love of baking she passed on to me. If Alice were still with us today, I know she would be proud to know her legacy continues through me and my children, Abigail, Mimi, and Eli.

It wasn't until I was an adult and had moved out of the house that I recognized the correlation between the food I grew up eating and the memories of my childhood, and realized how both of these things kept me emotionally connected to people, places, and events. Particular dishes have been like snapshots in my life journal, helping me to remember more fondly the details of time spent with family and friends.

My children often request their favorite dishes. If Abigail had her wish, we would eat Thai chicken and peanut sauce every night. Mimi loves my thumbprint jam scones, which I can't blame her for because I love them too! Eli is still too young to tell me what his favorite dish is, but I can assure you the boy loves to help me bake, and then to eat whatever we've made together.

I love thinking about my children making these dishes for their own friends and families someday, and perhaps even preparing them for me. But for now, I continue to cook and bake with them as much as I can, hoping to instill the same passion my mom and Alice instilled in me.

Since I used to own a wedding cake decorating business, my kids are accustomed to having homemade cupcakes and custom cakes to celebrate their birthdays. Both girls take party planning very seriously; deciding on the type of cake and how it will be decorated is a big deal. Abigail loves planning her menu with her favorite dishes, while Mimi insists on doing most of the decorating on her own.

All year long we celebrate accomplishments, large and small, with food. When Abigail competed in her first soccer game in second grade, we came home and baked chocolate chip cookies to commemorate a game well played. We did the same for Mimi when she was four years old and the only girl on the T-ball team.

I love my husband's anticipation as his birthday approaches. Rob will drop subtle hints about how much he loves banana cream pie—my banana cream pie, to be precise. These moments are what life is all about: being together as we laugh, live, and love with our favorite foods at the table.

Most days find me in my car driving the kids to and from school, friends' houses, sports practices, and other activities. By the time I get home I'm exhausted. When I cook I try to keep everything as simple as possible without compromising flavor or quality. Because of our hectic schedules, the way I cook often incorporates shortcuts and ingredients I have on hand, or that are readily available at my local supermarket. As much as I enjoy cooking, on most nights I don't want to spend a lot of time in the

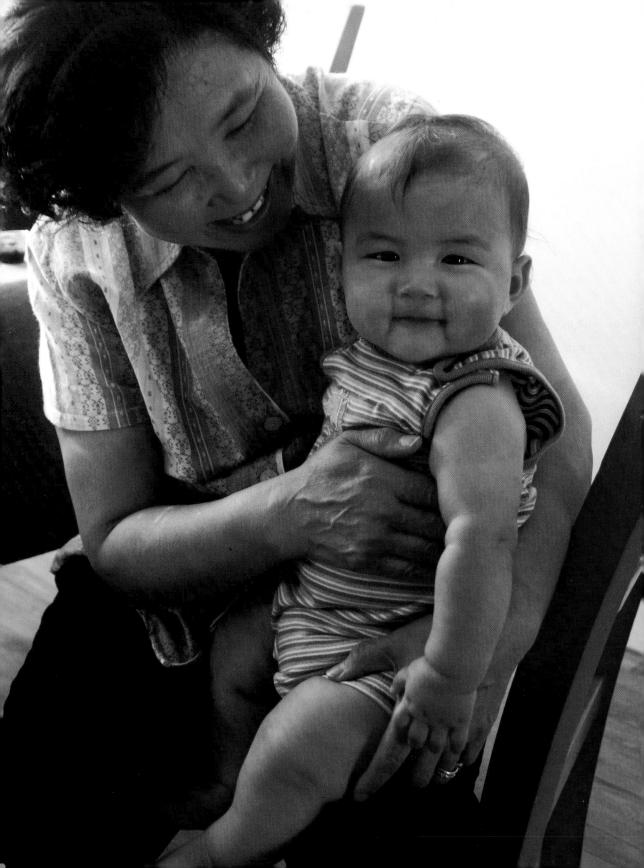

kitchen. Instead, I would rather pull a delicious meal together quickly and spend the rest of the time listening to my family talk about their day.

I know the food I prepare throughout the years will have a lasting impact on all three of my children long after they leave the house. Just like my mother's, the dishes I cook are simple, easy to prepare, and do not require special culinary know-how. However, each dish is delicious from the first bite to the last. Good food doesn't need to be complicated in order for it to be unforgettable. Some of the best and most-requested dishes I make for my family and friends use only a few ingredients.

This simple approach to food is the same philosophy behind my food blog, Savory Sweet Life.

It's my sincere desire that the recipes in this book will become your new family favorites to celebrate both everyday and special occasions. Whether you're warming up with a hot cup of cocoa on a blustery December day or are in need of a refreshing treat to keep you cool during the summer, the food from this book will help you benchmark the good stuff in life for years to come.

## THE STORY OF SAVORY SWEET LIFE

I'll never forget the night Savory Sweet Life was born. The girls were fast asleep in their beds, and I could hear Rob snoring on the other side of the house. With a pint of coffee-flavored ice cream to keep me company, I held Eli in one arm and checked my e-mails with the other. It was February and another month had gone by since I had made my New Year's resolution to start a blog. After many late nights feeding Eli and contemplating the type of blog I wanted to write, I decided it would be fun to document the process of recipes from start to finish from the perspective of a home cook. This would also give me a chance to flex my photography skills and share my love of cooking. So that night, I created Savory Sweet Life. The next day I posted my first recipe, for Mango Pico de Gallo.

I started blogging to have a creative outlet just for myself. I was new to the blogging phenomenon and wasn't sure what to expect or whether I was doing it correctly. So I just decided to photograph, write, and share what I wanted, and without any expectations. Blogging became a cheap form of therapy, and helped me enjoy my kids and husband more. By the end of the day, after devoting all my energy to my family, I was able to do something for me, and this made me a happier and more fulfilled mother and wife. When everyone went to bed, those late-night hours were mine to do what I wanted, with only the hum of the dryer in the background. I looked forward to working on Savory Sweet Life every night in the quiet of the house.

Even though very few people visited my site initially, I didn't care. I just enjoyed the process. I plugged myself into the food community using social media—mainly Twitter—and I loved making new friends who also enjoyed sharing what they were cooking and eating at home. It wasn't very long before Savory Sweet Life started getting noticed by respected websites, including Martha's Circle, a network of blogs chosen by the editors of *Martha Stewart Living*. Forbes.com also named me as one of the very best food bloggers, and in the same month I won *Saveur*'s cover photo contest. Before long I was writing for PBS Parents, contributing regularly to The Pioneer Woman's TastyKitchen.com, and writing this book.

To this day, I reflect on how crazy this all is and how incredibly grateful I am to the readership of Savory Sweet Life. I'm also thankful to my food-loving friends who have supported me and continue to do so on this journey.

What started out as a creative outlet has become a purpose-driven life, and I thank God for it daily.

## HOW TO USE THIS BOOK

Cooking for family and friends is a joy for me. I love when people come over and stay for hours, when we can spend time catching up with each other over good food and conversation. I've never been one who plans set menus or decorates the dining table with elaborate floral centerpieces, coordinating dishware, and complementary stemmed glassware. In fact, I don't own any delicate china. Most of the time when we throw parties we use mismatched plates, cups, utensils, and a collection of eclectic serving dishes. For me, it has never been about hosting the picture-perfect party. It's about creating a warm and inviting environment where guests feel welcome and my family and I can enjoy the evening with very little stress.

## About the Photography in This Book

I've loved photography since I was a little kid. Photos to me are like visual stories to help us remember our loved ones and document our lives. I bought my first digital point-and-shoot in 2001, right before my daughter Abigail was born. It felt so amazing to be able to shoot a gazillion photos and delete the ones I didn't want! The following year I purchased a digital DSLR and started to take photography more seriously. By the time I started my blog, I was on my second DSLR and shooting food felt very natural for me.

Savory Sweet Life has always been a documentary-style food site. It was an unexpected blessing not only to write this cookbook, but to do all the food photography as well. When you see the photos in this book, I want you to feel as if you are in the kitchen with me and we're cooking these easy, delicious, approachable recipes together.

If you're a visual learner like I am, you're going to love this cookbook. The photos are intended to help take the intimidation out of cooking and inspire you to prepare memorable, good food for your family and friends all year long.

This cookbook is divided into chapters inspired by everyday life moments that occur throughout the year. Although each chapter contains a set of recipes, the chapters themselves are not menus. Recipes are grouped together to provide inspiration for a particular occasion, but depending on your needs, you may want to make one or two or all of them. Use the recipes in this book in a way that makes sense to you, creating traditions and memories with the people you love.

## MY FAVORITE THINGS

I'll always remember the day when Rob and I arrived at Macy's for the prewedding ritual known as registering for gifts. The sheer thrill of carrying an electronic scanning gun around the kitchen department turned me into a kid in a candy store, except that I was a kid pre-fueled with a double tall latte. Rob couldn't have cared less what we registered for, but he delighted in my excitement as I marveled at all the gadgets and appliances with grand hopes of cooking for us as a married couple and perhaps as a family someday.

About ten minutes into the whole experience, a sense of panic came over me. I wasn't prepared for how overwhelming it would be to decide what we actually needed compared to what we really, really wanted. With every item, I mentally romanticized how we'd use it together in the kitchen to justify adding it to the registry. Needless to say, if we had it to do over again I'd have left the ice cream malt shake maker off our list. For the record, we never did use the shake maker and sold it at a yard sale a couple of years ago for $2, brand new.

However, we did manage to register for some items that at the time seemed unnecessary and indulgent, but ended up being very practical for everyday cooking.

Here's a list of my favorite kitchen tools that truly make life easier. If I had to scan items for my wedding registry all over again, these are the ones I'd choose. Some of them represent a financial investment, but they're worth every penny if you cook regularly.

- **Stand mixer** A good stand mixer is worth its weight in gold. Mine is twelve years old and it's still going strong. Although they aren't cheap, I've calculated that my stand mixer has cost 5¢ a day over the years I've owned it, with that amount decreasing as time goes by. If you look at it as an investment, it will pay itself off and make life—especially baking—so much more enjoyable. Truthfully, there's nothing else quite like it.

- **An electric hand mixer** is also a great tool—a notch below a stand mixer but several steps above having to mix by hand. With starting prices around $20 (sometimes less), they're perfect for those who bake only occasionally.

- **Food processor** I own a mini 4-cup food processor, also known as a mini-prep chopper. This clever tool saves me so much time dicing and chopping—I couldn't imagine not owning one. My favorite use for my mini-chopper is mincing garlic and chopping onions, my least favorite activities to do by hand. And there's a bonus: no onion tears.

- **Cookie scoops** If you bake cookies or cupcakes with any frequency, a cookie scoop is a must-have. This inexpensive tool makes me look like a pro baker by giving me uniform cookies, cupcakes, and muffins, and beautiful ice cream scoops. They usually come in three sizes: small, medium (my favorite), and large.

- **Disposable pastry bags and a selection of cake tips** If you love baking cupcakes or decorating cakes to celebrate special occasions, disposable pastry bags and a few cake tips will serve you well. Bags are usually around 25¢ each and tips $1. I recommend having a dozen bags and at the very least one star tip. The bags and star tip will give you nice decorative borders for beautiful-looking cakes.

- **Rimmed baking sheets** Baking sheets are not only practical, they are also multitasking kitchen necessities. Whether you're baking a pizza, cake, or cookies or roasting vegetables and meats, rimmed baking sheets will make cleanup easier and also protect your oven from excessive spillage. If you can, stock your kitchen with at least two of the same kind. They'll stack nicely and take up less space in your cabinet.

- **Parchment paper** Baking with parchment paper makes life so much less stressful, especially when it comes to cakes and cookies. I never have to worry about batter sticking to pans, and my cakes never get stuck when I invert them (a baker's worst nightmare). And using parchment paper makes cleaning up a cinch. I like to crumple up the parchment paper when I'm done and recycle it, with very little pan washing to do later.

- **Sharp chef's knife** Only in the last couple of years did I fully "get" why having at least one sharp chef's knife is important for home cooks. The first time I ever used a quality chef's knife, I was amazed at how easy it was to cut different types of meats, vegetables, and fruits. Cutting was suddenly a nonissue, exactly what it should be.

- **Kitchen shears** Having one pair of kitchen shears is great, but owning two pairs is even better, because they get so much use that one set is always sitting in the dishwasher waiting to be washed. They're great for cutting parchment paper, snipping uncooked bacon into bits, cutting lettuce for salad, trimming stems from a bouquet of flowers, and a plethora of other things. They're my most useful and beloved kitchen utensil of all.

- **Pots and pans** If you ask any professional chef, they'll let you in on a little secret: Don't bother buying complete sets of cookware. Instead, buy individual pieces based on their performance. I personally love having a stainless steel saucepan, a nonstick skillet, and a cast-iron skillet/grill pan. I'm indifferent to pots. As long as it has a lid, I'm happy. Having a Dutch oven isn't essential, but it's a very nice heavy-duty pot to have on hand.

- **Bakeware** Unless you're planning on baking tiered cakes often, two 8-inch or 9-inch cake pans are all you'll need for baking birthday or other special-occasion cakes. I also recommend having Bundt and loaf pans, a 9 x 13-inch baking dish, an 8-inch square casserole dish, a pie plate, a ceramic tart pan, and both mini and regular-size muffin tins.

## Herb Container Gardens

Although my father was a prolific gardener, apparently I did not inherit his green thumb. In fact, my success rate at growing vegetables is too embarrassing to reveal.

But years ago I decided to make a container garden of the herbs I use the most in cooking. I was motivated by practical reasons, such as how expensive fresh herbs are, but I also loved the idea of snipping off just enough stems or leaves to use in a dish or as a garnish. Fresh herbs add wonderful flavor to dishes and make them look special.

I also discovered that herbs are one of the simplest groups of plants to cultivate, which was an extra incentive for me to give container gardening a try. Herbs don't require a lot of space, are very easy to take care of, and add a nice splash of color to your porch, stairs, deck, patio, balcony, or window ledge from spring through fall.

Before you start planting, decide which herbs you'll likely cook with the most often. My top three favorite herbs to grow are basil, thyme, and mint. Other herbs I recommend for a container garden are rosemary, oregano, sage, parsley, cilantro, chives, and dill.

Because herbs love sunshine, choose a location outside that gets at least 5 hours of full sun a day. Determine how much space you can allow for either a big container or several smaller ones, depending on how many herbs you plan on planting. Once you have an idea of how you'll utilize the space, look through any pots you may already own or go shopping for new ones to fulfill your creative vision. The best choice is containers that have drainage holes for watering, such as terra-cotta pots.

Next, go to your local garden center or nursery and select your herbs. I recommend starters over seeds so you can begin cultivating your fresh herbs immediately. You'll also want to purchase a bag of good potting soil for your herbs to thrive in.

To plant your herbs, fill a container loosely with soil until it's 2 to 3 inches from the top. Remove the herb plants from their containers and loosen each root ball with your fingers. Decide where you would like to plant each herb, and then take a small trowel or use your hands to scoop a hole large enough to accommodate the plant. Make sure to leave enough space between the plants to give them space to grow. Carefully fill the space around each herb with fresh soil and gently pat the soil down. Give your new garden a nice drink of water. Great job—you're now growing your own herbs!

Don't forget to water your herbs regularly. You want to water them just enough to keep the soil moist but not drenched.

- **Blender** From making smoothies and cocktails to pureeing soups and sauces, a good blender will make time spent in the kitchen more enjoyable by doing a multitude of tasks in a short amount of time.

- **Rice cooker** If making perfect rice every time is important to you, a rice cooker is a must-have appliance. Rice cookers come in all shapes and sizes; choose one according to how much rice your family will consume in any given meal. My favorite size is a 5-cup rice cooker—large enough to feed my family and small enough to store in a kitchen cabinet.

- **Slow cooker and pressure cooker** Both of these timeless kitchen appliances are great to have for one-pot meals. Slow cookers are ideal for anyone who loves to start dinner early in the morning and forget about it until it's time to eat. Pressure cookers are handy for saving time on cooking certain types of dishes that would typically take hours: braising meat or cooking a beef stew can take less than an hour without compromising flavor or texture.

# one

# SUNDAY MORNINGS

Sunday mornings are special around here. I love to get up early to make my family a warm breakfast before they wake up. I quietly leave my comfy bed, put on my brown fleece robe, and head for the kitchen. As I listen to the familiar sound of roasted coffee beans grinding (music to my ears), I focus my attention on what to bake for breakfast.

After taking a quick inventory of the ingredients I have on hand, I preheat the oven and put my stand mixer to work. Butter, sugar, eggs, and flour come together for what will become a delicious coffee cake. I find it peaceful to drink my coffee next to the radiant heat from the oven with the sweet scent of cake filling the air.

My second daughter, Mimi, discovered my Sunday-morning routine and often joins me for a special time of baking together. She drinks her tea and I drink my coffee. Together we bake and keep each other company.

Once breakfast is ready, Mimi runs through the house to wake everyone up. "Breakfast is ready . . . come on! Mom and I made muffins!" she hollers, shaking Rob until he finally gets out of bed.

When we're all sitting at the table, I pause to enjoy the moment—all of us together without feeling the typical weekday rush. This is what makes Sundays special. Seeing the eagerness on the faces of my family as they're about to dig into breakfast makes the early rise worthwhile.

# Cinnamon Coffee Cake Muffins

Any morning that begins with one of these muffins and a cup of hot coffee is off to a great start—and the whole house will smell of warm coffee cake goodness.

CRUMB TOPPING

½ cup all-purpose flour

4 tablespoons (½ stick) cold unsalted butter, cubed

¼ cup granulated sugar

¼ cup firmly packed light or dark brown sugar

1½ teaspoons ground cinnamon

¼ teaspoon salt

MUFFINS

1¼ cups granulated sugar

8 tablespoons (1 stick) unsalted butter

3 eggs

1 cup sour cream

1 teaspoon pure vanilla extract

1 teaspoon ground cinnamon

¼ teaspoon salt

2 teaspoons baking powder

2 cups all-purpose flour

1. Preheat the oven to 400°F. Spray a generous amount of nonstick spray into a crumbled paper towel and grease the top of a 12-cup muffin tin. Line the tin with 12 paper baking cups.

2. To make the crumb topping, combine the flour, butter, sugar, brown sugar, cinnamon, and salt in a food processor and pulse until the mixture resembles large coarse crumbs. (If you don't have a food processor, use a pastry blender or two knives to cut the butter with the other ingredients.) Set the topping aside.

3. Prepare the batter: Using a hand or stand mixer, cream the sugar and butter together on medium speed for 3 minutes, until light and fluffy. Add the eggs one at a time, waiting for each egg to be mixed in before adding another. Add the sour cream, vanilla, cinnamon, and salt, and mix until the sour cream is combined. Reduce the mixer speed to low and add the baking powder and flour. Mix until the batter is smooth, about 2 minutes. It will be very thick.

4. Place about 2 tablespoons of the batter into each muffin cup. Spread the batter with a spoon so the bottom of each cup is covered. Sprinkle 1 generous tablespoon of the crumb topping on top of the batter, followed by 2 more tablespoons

of batter. Finish each muffin with 1 tablespoon of crumb topping. Don't worry if the batter is slightly higher than the muffin tin.

5. Bake the muffins for 12 minutes. Then reduce the oven temperature to 350°F and bake for 13 minutes more, or until the center of a muffin springs back when touched.

6. Allow the muffins to rest in the tin for 10 minutes before carefully releasing them from the tin.

*Cook's note:* These muffins can be stored in a zip-top bag in the freezer. Set them on the counter for 30 minutes to thaw before serving.

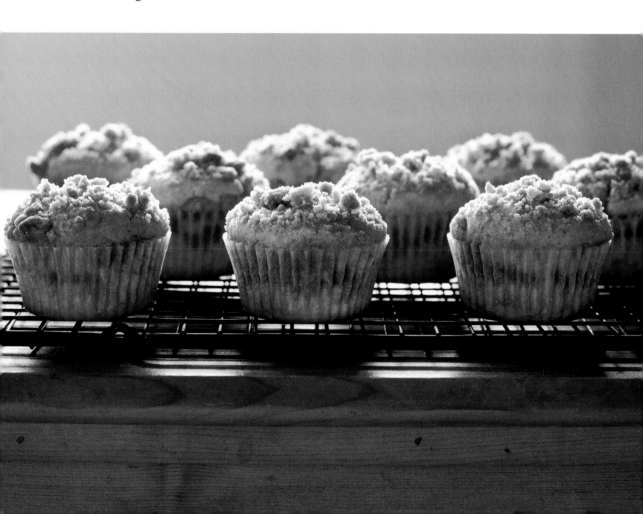

# Spinach Ricotta Quiche

I'm a big fan of quiche. It makes a perfect meal—not just for breakfast, but for lunch or dinner too. Using eggs, cream, and cheese as a base, I love to add a leafy vegetable like spinach. But you can be as creative as you like with quiche—the possible additions are almost limitless. Leftovers also heat up beautifully in the microwave.

**MAKES 1 QUICHE;
SERVES 8**

**One unbaked 9-inch
pie crust (store-bought
or homemade)**

**4 eggs**

**1 cup heavy cream**

**1 cup ricotta cheese**

**1 cup grated sharp
cheddar cheese**

**½ teaspoon kosher salt**

**½ teaspoon freshly
ground black pepper**

**2 cups fresh spinach,
cooked, chopped,
and all excess water
squeezed out**

1. Preheat the oven to 375°F. Spray a 9-inch pie plate or tart pan with nonstick spray.

2. Place the pie crust in the plate and gently pat it down around the base and sides. Crimp the outside edges of the crust or cut the excess off with a knife. Using a fork, poke several holes in the pie crust.

3. In a medium bowl, whisk the eggs, cream, ricotta, cheddar, salt, and pepper until everything is well combined.

4. Evenly distribute the cooked spinach in the pie crust. Pour in the egg mixture, filling the plate up to ¼ inch from the top.

5. Bake for 40 to 45 minutes, or until the center of the quiche is firm when pressed. Allow the quiche to cool for 5 to 10 minutes before serving.

*Just for fun:* Add 1 cup crumbled cooked bacon, diced ham, or chopped cooked sausage.

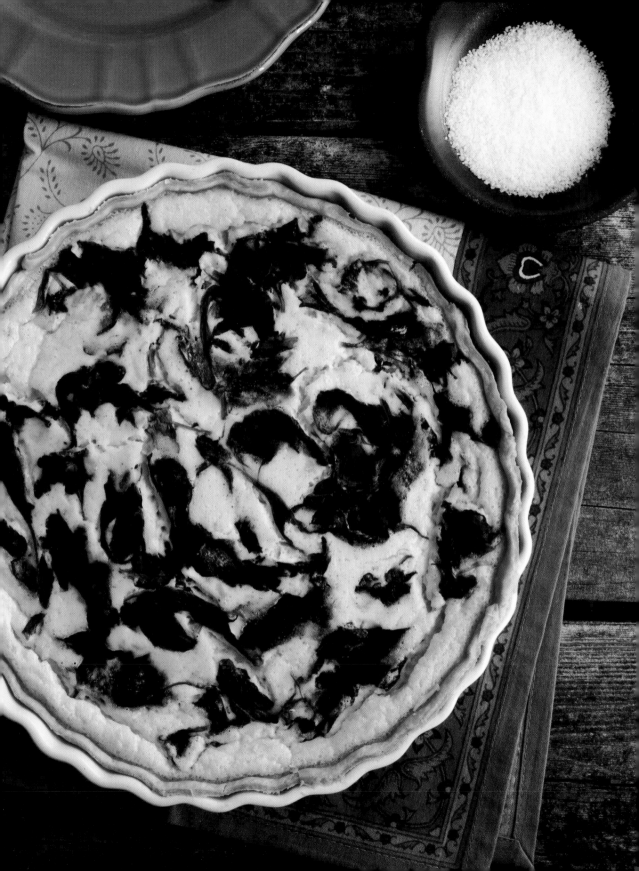

# Peach Croissants

I love recipes that require minimal effort but yield impressive results. These peach croissants are exactly that. Using premade puff pastry sheets, a peach, and a bit of sugar and cinnamon, you end up with a bakerylike pastry that smells and tastes absolutely divine. When people ask me for the recipe, I always feel a little guilty. Most of the time they ask, "That was it?" Yep, that was it.

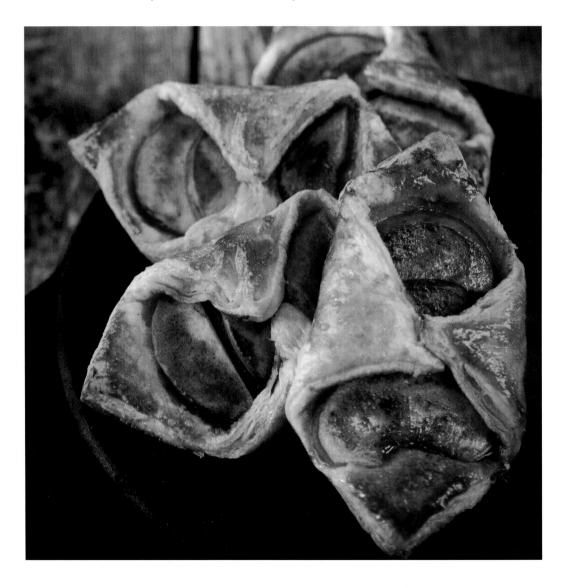

1. Preheat the oven to 375°F, and line a baking sheet with parchment paper.

2. Cut the peach in half and remove the pit. Slice each peach half into 6 slices. In a small bowl, mix the sugar and cinnamon together. Set aside.

3. Roll the puff pastry sheet slightly larger than actual size on a lightly floured surface. Cut the sheet in half vertically and then horizontally so you have 4 equal square pieces. Rotate a square of puff pastry so it looks like a diamond. Place 3 peach slices across the center of the diamond from left to right. Sprinkle one-fourth of the cinnamon-sugar mixture evenly over the peach slices. Grab the top and bottom corners and bring them to the center, pinching them together to seal them. Repeat this process with each of the remaining squares.

4. Place the croissants on the baking sheet. Brush the puff pastry with the egg wash. Bake for 25 minutes, or until the croissants are golden brown.

*Just for fun:* Immediately after you remove the peach croissants from the oven, brush each one with simple syrup (¼ cup water and ¼ cup sugar cooked for 3 minutes over medium heat) to give it a nice glossy sheen, just like the professional bakeries. Or sprinkle each croissant with a dusting of confectioners' sugar.

*Variations:* Plums, nectarines, peeled apples, and pears work just as well. You can also use canned peaches if fresh ones are out of season—just be sure to use the ones that are packed in their own juice. Rinse the canned peaches off and pat them dry as best as you can before using them.

1 fresh peach

2 tablespoons granulated sugar

2 teaspoons ground cinnamon

1 sheet frozen puff pastry, thawed

Egg wash: 1 egg yolk beaten with 1 teaspoon water

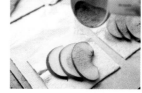

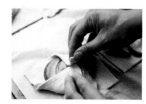

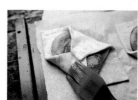

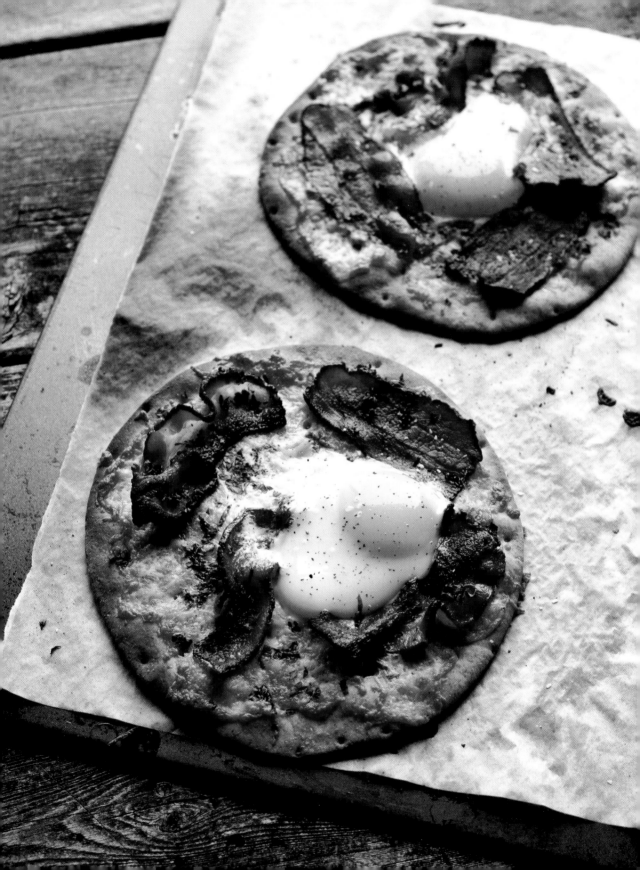

# Breakfast Pizza

Pizza for breakfast? You bet! My kids love eggs and toast for breakfast, and they also love cheese pizza. One morning I had a "lightbulb" idea and combined their two favorite foods into one savory dish. Needless to say, it has become a staple in our home. Sometimes we even eat it for lunch or dinner!

1. Preheat the oven to 500°F.

2. Brush the olive oil over each side of the pita breads. Place the pitas on a large baking sheet, and sprinkle the cheese evenly over them. Arrange 4 bacon halves around the outside edge of each pita. Crack an egg in the center of each pita. sprinkle parsley or scallions on top of each pizza.

3. Bake for 8 minutes. (If the egg white is still not completely cooked, place the baking sheet under the broiler on the low setting: Cook for 1 or 2 minutes, or until the egg whites are no longer runny.)

*Variations:* Substitute crumbled cooked sausage, ham, or vegetarian meat substitute for the bacon. Add other toppings such as sliced tomatoes, mushrooms, and/or olives.

**SERVES 4**

Extra-virgin olive oil

4 pieces whole wheat flat pita bread (not pita pockets)

One 8-ounce package Italian blend shredded cheese (mozzarella, Parmesan, Provolone)

8 bacon slices, cooked and cut in half

4 eggs

¼ cup chopped fresh parsley or green onions

# Chocolate Chocolate Chip Banana Bread

Did you know that the secret to making great banana bread is using those dark, speckled, overripe, squishy bananas that are usually tossed out? It's true. Overripe bananas are sweeter and more flavorful than fresher, beautiful (less ripe) ones. Add some cocoa powder, sour cream, and chocolate chips and you have rich, moist, chocolate banana bread that will keep you from tossing out those overripe bananas ever again.

**MAKES 1 LOAF
(18 SLICES)**

8 tablespoons (1 stick) unsalted butter, at room temperature

½ cup granulated sugar

1 egg

1 teaspoon pure vanilla extract

2 large very ripe bananas, mashed

½ cup sour cream

1 cup all-purpose flour

2 tablespoons unsweetened cocoa powder

1 teaspoon baking soda

¼ teaspoon salt

1 cup mini chocolate chips

1. Preheat the oven to 350°F. Generously grease a 9 x 5-inch loaf pan with nonstick spray, and set it aside.

2. In a large bowl or the bowl of a stand mixer, cream the butter and sugar together on medium-high speed for 3 minutes, until nice and fluffy. Beat in the egg, vanilla, bananas, and sour cream. Mixing on medium speed, slowly add the flour, cocoa powder, baking soda, and salt. Mix for 2 minutes, or until the batter looks smooth. Scrape down the sides and bottom of the bowl and mix for an additional minute. Remove from the mixer and stir in the chocolate chips until well combined.

3. Pour the batter into the loaf pan. Bake for 50 minutes, or until done (see below).

4. Allow the bread to cool in the pan for 15 minutes. Then, to release the bread, slowly and carefully run a butter knife along the sides of the pan. Grab the sides of the pan and gently shake it up and down and side to side to loosen the bread before inverting it onto a wire rack to cool.

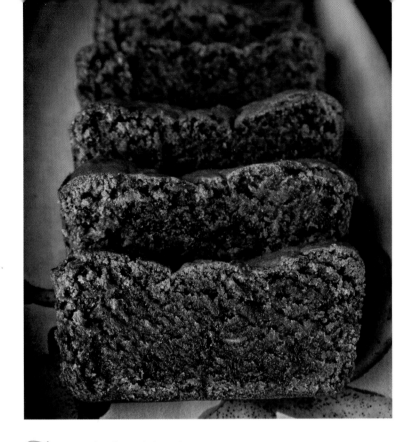

*Testing the bread for doneness:* Stick a wood skewer into the center of the bread and remove it quickly. If the stick is free of batter, the bread is completely baked. If any batter is pulled up, bake the bread for 5 minutes longer and test again.

*Avoiding disaster:* Do not let the bread cool in the pan for longer than 15 minutes after removing it from the oven. Otherwise the bread will adhere to the sides of the pan, making it difficult to remove.

*Freezing ripe bananas:* Unpeeled overripe bananas can be frozen in plastic bags. When you are ready to use them, thaw the bananas on the counter for one hour. The bananas will be mushy—just perfect for making banana bread.

# Overnight Baked French Toast Casserole

I love breakfast recipes in which most of the preparation is done the night before, so when morning comes, all you have to do is put it in the oven. This bread-pudding-like casserole is a great choice when family and friends come to stay with us, or when I want to use up a day-old loaf of French bread.

**SERVES 6 TO 8**

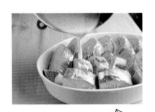

**FRENCH TOAST**

1 loaf French bread
(standard, not a
baguette), cut into
1½-inch-thick slices

6 large eggs

2 cups half-and-half

2 teaspoons pure
vanilla extract

½ teaspoon ground
cinnamon

**TOPPING**

1 cup (2 sticks) unsalted
butter

½ cup firmly packed
light brown sugar

½ cup pure maple
syrup

¼ teaspoon kosher salt

1 cup Candied Pecans
(page 217), chopped

1. Generously coat a 9 x 13-inch baking dish with nonstick spray or butter. Arrange the bread in the dish in overlapping slices.

2. In a large bowl, beat together the eggs, half-and-half, vanilla, and cinnamon. Pour this egg mixture evenly over the bread slices. Cover the baking dish with plastic wrap or foil, and refrigerate overnight or for at least 3 hours.

3. The next morning, remove the baking dish from the refrigerator. Preheat the oven to 350°F.

4. To make the topping, combine the butter, brown sugar, maple syrup, and salt in a small saucepan over medium heat. Stir until the mixture begins to bubble and foam. Once the butter has melted, slowly pour the mixture over the bread and in between the slices.

5. Bake, uncovered, for 40 to 45 minutes, until golden on top. Remove the baking dish from the oven. Baste the top of the casserole with the maple syrup sauce and top with the chopped pecans before serving.

*For grown-ups only:* I like to add 2 tablespoons of bourbon (whiskey) when cooking the maple syrup sauce to make this breakfast really special.

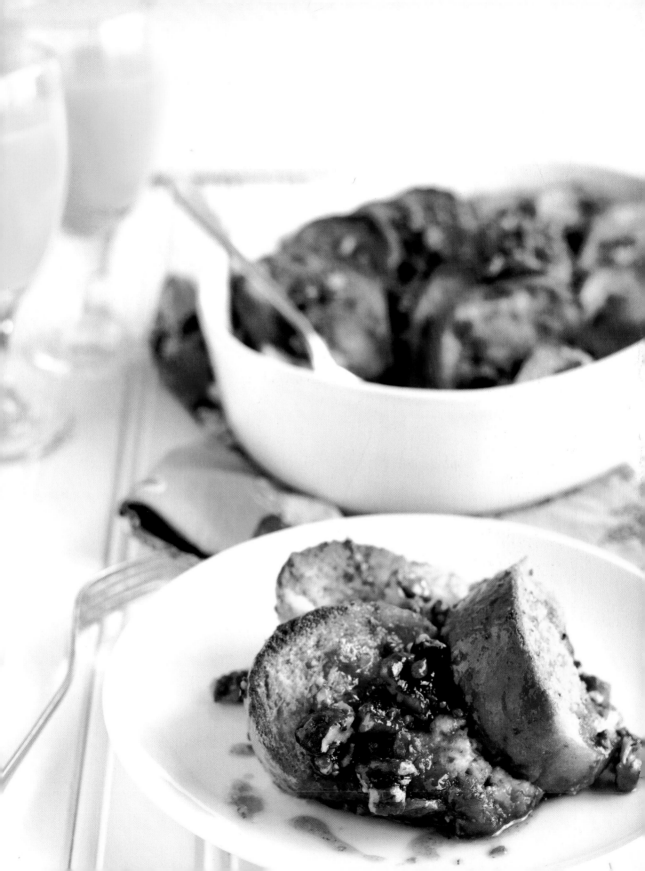

# two

# MOTHER'S DAY BREAKFAST IN BED

Dear Rob,

   As you know, Mother's Day is approaching quickly. In fact, it's next Sunday and I wanted to remind you—a week early—to save you the trouble of running over to the drugstore that morning, hoping you'll find a card that articulates what a wonderful mom I've been to our three children. I know the kids will be making me homemade cards, which I absolutely love. But what I want from you is not a card. Instead, I would like at least one (preferably all) of the ideas I'm about to share with you.

**1. Let me sleep in.** To be able to wake up as late as I want would be awesome. Since this rarely happens, I'd appreciate it more than you could ever know. What this means for you, darling husband, is waking up when the kids wake up and making sure they understand that I'm not to be disturbed until I've decided to come out of my sleeping chamber.

**2. Feed the family.** I'd enjoy sleeping in more if I knew the kids were being fed and a cup of hot coffee was waiting for me as soon as I was able to join you at the table. If you're feeding the kids anyway, breakfast in bed would be wonderful (hint hint, wink wink). I've set out a few of my favorite recipes to help you choose: a blueberry oat smoothie, Nutella banana crêpes, or smoked salmon bagels, honey-mint fruit salad, perfect scrambled eggs, roasted potatoes, and brown sugar bacon.

**3. Clean up.** After the kids have barged into our bedroom because they couldn't wait for me to get up to wish me a happy Mother's Day, it would be nice to know that a pile of dirty dishes isn't waiting for me in the kitchen sink.

**4. Repeat steps 2 and 3** for lunch and dinner.

If you insist on getting me a gift, may I suggest the gift of time? It's free and means more to me than adding the latest World's Greatest Mom mug to my growing collection of Happy Mother's Day dishware. Free time allows me to do whatever I want all day long without having to lift a finger. If you want bonus points, washing and vacuuming the car, paying particular attention to the Cheerios underneath the seats and in hard-to-reach places, would really make this Mother's Day the second-best present ever.

Love,
Alice

PS: I wouldn't stop you from getting me a gift certificate for a pedicure . . . just saying.

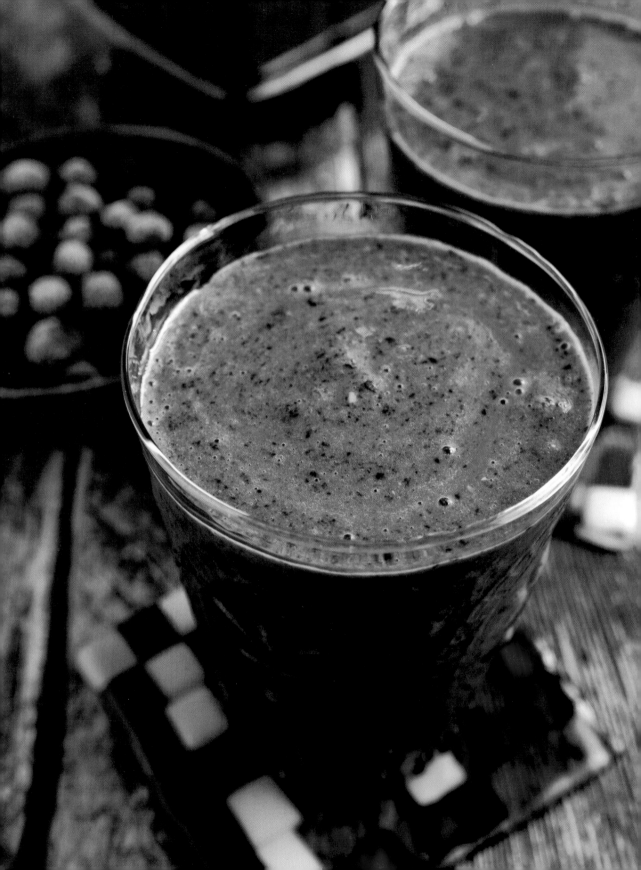

# Blueberry Oat Smoothie

Mornings around our house can be quite hectic. The kids are scrambling to get ready for school and I'm doing what I can to help them. This often leaves little time for breakfast, which isn't a very good way to start the day. I love smoothies because they can be made very quickly and the family can drink them on the go. And the best part of all: they're super healthy!

Put all the ingredients in a blender and blend until smooth.

*Not sweet enough?* Feel free to add a bit of your favorite sweetener to your smoothie. I might use white grape juice concentrate, agave syrup, honey, Sucralose (Splenda), or sugar.

**SERVES 1 OR 2**

**1 cup frozen blueberries**

**¼ cup rolled oats**

**½ banana**

**½ cup vanilla yogurt**

**1 cup milk**

**1 tablespoon vanilla whey protein powder (optional)**

# Honey-Mint Fruit Salad

If you can chop, you can look like a gourmet chef with this refreshing fruit salad tossed in a honey-mint dressing that accentuates each fruit's natural sweetness. This fruit salad is perfect for any occasion from casual to more formal get-togethers. In fact, it is the only fruit salad recipe you'll ever need!

**SERVES 6**

**Juice of 1 lime**

**3 tablespoons honey**

**3 tablespoons finely chopped fresh mint**

**6 to 8 cups cut-up mixed fresh fruit (see suggestions), in bite-size pieces**

In a large bowl, whisk the lime juice, honey, and mint until well combined. Add the fresh fruit and toss gently until the fruit is coated with the dressing.

*Fresh fruit suggestions:* Strawberries, blueberries, peaches, mangoes, pineapple, grapes, apples, pears, honeydew melon, cantaloupe, bananas, oranges, kiwis, and blackberries. My favorite combo is strawberries, blueberries, peaches, and kiwis.

*Time-saving tip:* Grocery stores sell fresh fruit platters. Use the precut fruit from these platters for this salad.

*Just for fun:* Add 2 tablespoons poppy seeds to the dressing for a noticeable and special added touch.

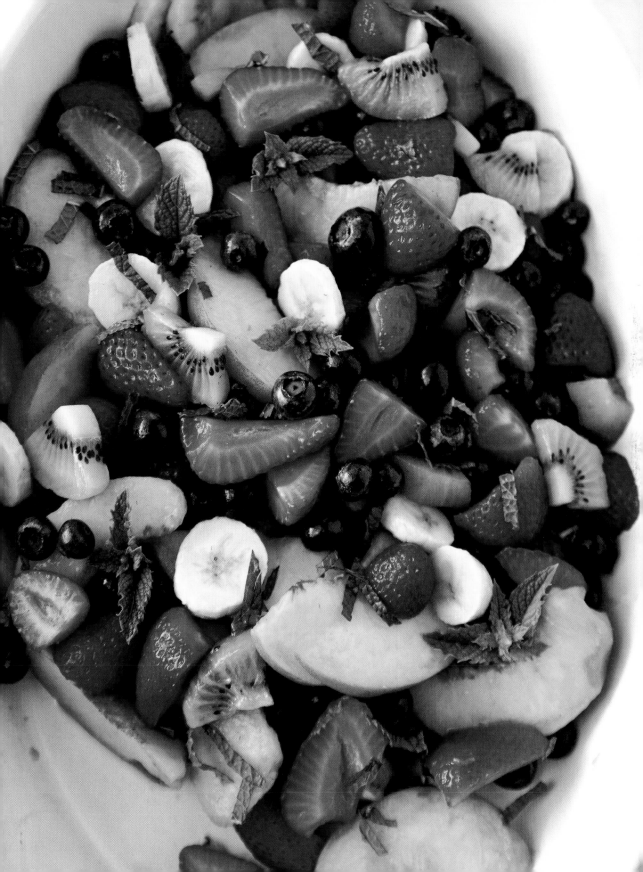

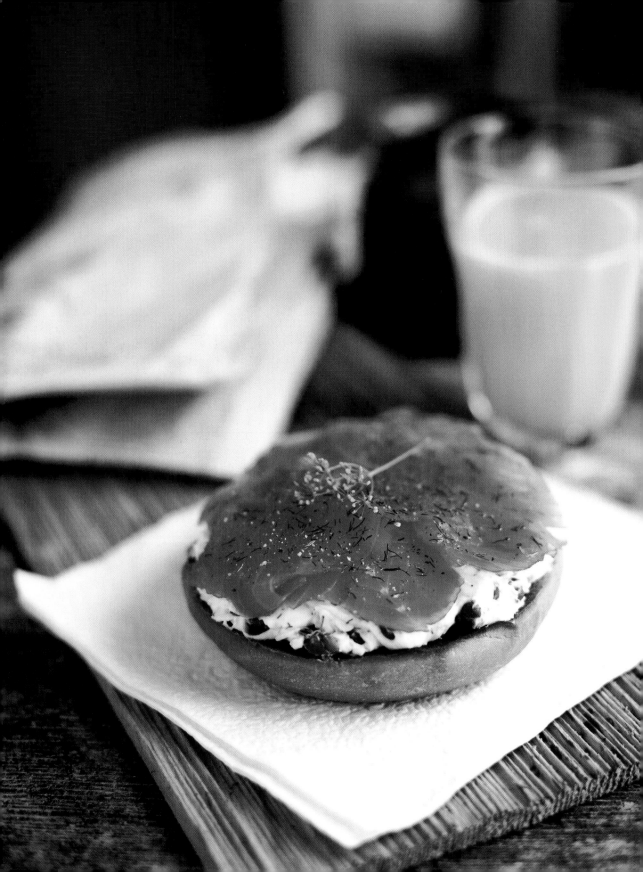

# Bagels with Smoked Salmon and Capers

I love the simplicity of this bold-tasting sandwich—biting into thin layers of smoked salmon with the creaminess of the cream cheese and the zing of the capers is such a treat. The crispy outer layer of a toasted bagel and the chewy bread inside are the perfect complement to this sandwich's flavorful ingredients.

In a bowl, combine the cream cheese and capers. Spread the cream cheese mixture equally over each toasted bagel half. Top each bagel off with the smoked salmon and a sprinkling of dill.

*Smaller serving sizes:* Use mini bagels for smaller portions—perfect for brunches, bridal and baby showers, or any gathering.

**MAKES 6 OPEN-FACED SANDWICHES**

**One 8-ounce package cream cheese, at room temperature**

**¼ cup capers, drained**

**3 plain bagels, split and toasted**

**One 8-ounce package sliced smoked salmon**

**1 teaspoon chopped fresh dill**

# Nutella, Strawberry, and Banana Crêpes

As much as I love eating Nutella straight from the jar, I also love cooking and baking with this addictive chocolate-hazelnut spread. My favorite combination with Nutella is bananas and strawberries inside these sweet vanilla crêpes, topped with a dollop of whipped cream or vanilla ice cream. Serve them for breakfast, brunch, or dessert and your family and friends will smile with joy.

**MAKES ABOUT 8 CRÊPES; SERVES 4 TO 6**

### CRÊPES

1 cup all-purpose flour

3 tablespoons granulated sugar

2 large eggs

1¼ cups whole milk

1 teaspoon pure vanilla extract

4 tablespoons (½ stick) unsalted butter, melted

### FILLING

1 cup Nutella

2 cups sliced fresh strawberries

3 bananas, sliced crosswise into ¼-inch-thick rounds

### TOPPING

¼ cup confectioners' sugar

Extra sliced strawberries and banana

¼ cup Nutella

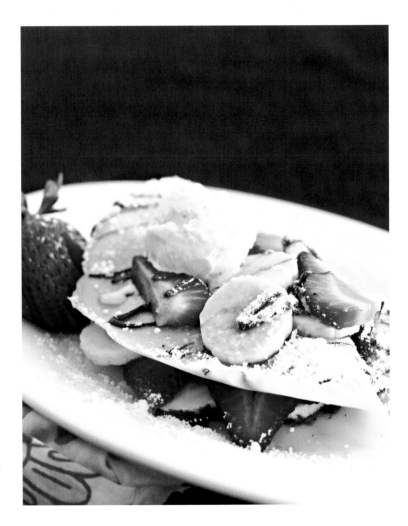

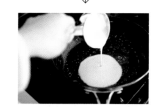

1. To make the crêpes, blend the flour, sugar, eggs, milk, and vanilla in a blender or food processor until the batter is smooth. Heat an 8-inch nonstick skillet over medium heat. Brush a generous coat of melted butter over the bottom and sides of the skillet. Pour ¼ cup of the batter into the center of the skillet, twirling your wrist in a circular motion so the batter spreads out evenly. Cook for 30 seconds, until the crêpe pulls away from the sides of the skillet. Gently flip the crêpe over with a rubber spatula, and cook for 5 seconds more. Remove the crêpe from the heat and transfer it to a plate. Repeat with the rest of the batter.

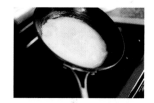

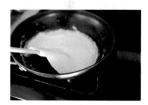

2. Spread a few tablespoons of Nutella over one side of each crêpe. Evenly place a few tablespoons of sliced strawberries and bananas on top of the Nutella. Fold the unfilled side of the crêpe over the filled side. Sprinkle with a dusting of confectioners' sugar and top it off with additional strawberries and bananas.

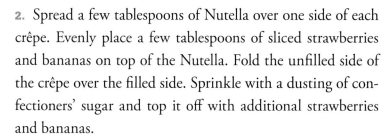

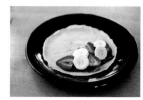

3. Finish the crêpes off by melting the ¼ cup Nutella in the microwave for 15 seconds and then drizzling it on top.

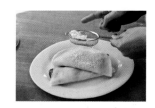

*Just for fun:* For an extra-special added touch, scoop a dollop of sweetened whipped cream or vanilla ice cream over each crêpe.

# Perfect Scrambled Eggs

I don't mess around when it comes to scrambled eggs. I like mine to be buttery, light, lightly salted, and not overcooked (evidenced by brown patches). Don't you? I have realized through the years, from several family members, that not everyone knows how to prepare this staple dish because they have never been properly taught. With a few tips, you'll be making perfect scrambled eggs every time.

**SERVES 4**

6 eggs

¼ cup half-and-half

2 tablespoons unsalted butter

Salt and freshly ground black pepper

1. In a medium bowl, whisk the eggs and half-and-half until lightly beaten.

2. In a large nonstick skillet, melt the butter over medium heat. Slowly pour the egg mixture into the skillet. When soft curds form, gently stir the eggs with a heat-resistant rubber spatula from one side of the skillet to the other, folding the eggs over themselves. When all the liquid has been cooked but the eggs still have a slightly wet sheen to them, immediately remove the skillet from the heat.

3. Season with salt and pepper to taste, and serve.

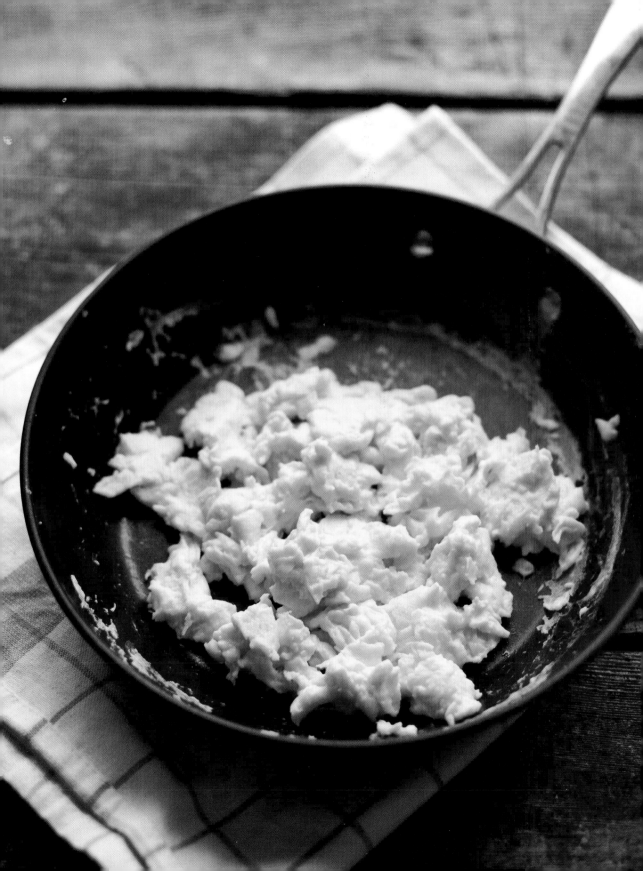

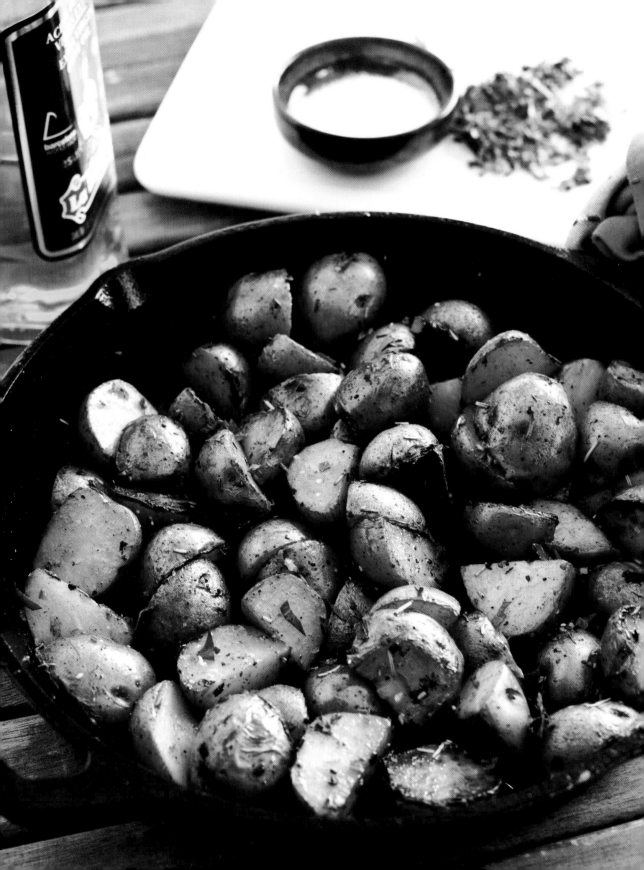

# Roasted Skillet Potatoes

My favorite all-American breakfast of pancakes and eggs is never complete without a side of warm seasoned potatoes. Preparing roasted potatoes in a cast-iron skillet imparts extra flavor and makes them the perfect side dish for breakfast or dinner.

1. In a medium bowl, combine 2 tablespoons of the vegetable oil with the salt, rosemary, thyme, garlic salt, and pepper. Add the potatoes and toss until they're coated with the oil and seasonings.

2. Heat the remaining ½ tablespoon vegetable oil in a large cast-iron skillet over medium-high heat. When the oil is shimmering but not smoking, add the potatoes. Cook the potatoes for 12 to 15 minutes, stirring them every few minutes, until they are browned and fork-tender.

*Variation:* If you love garlic, toss the roasted potatoes with 3 minced garlic cloves and 2 tablespoons chopped fresh parsley at the end.

**SERVES 4 TO 6**

**2½ tablespoons vegetable oil**

**1 teaspoon kosher salt**

**½ teaspoon dried rosemary**

**½ teaspoon dried thyme**

**½ teaspoon garlic salt**

**¼ teaspoon freshly ground black pepper**

**2 pounds baby red potatoes, scrubbed and quartered**

# Baked Brown Sugar Bacon

I've tried cooking bacon many different ways, but I've found that baking it produces the best results. It consistently has a better texture than you get from frying or from using the microwave. Adding a little bit of brown sugar before baking the bacon contributes just enough caramelized sweetness to create that addictive savory-sweet combination everyone loves.

**SERVES 4**

**1 pound quality thick-cut bacon**

**⅓ cup firmly packed light brown sugar**

1. Preheat the oven to 400°F. Place a wire rack on top of a rimmed baking sheet.

2. Toss the bacon slices with the brown sugar in a medium bowl. Lay the bacon slices on the wire rack and bake for 25 to 30 minutes, until crisp.

*Just for fun:* Stir ½ teaspoon cayenne pepper into the brown sugar for some added heat.

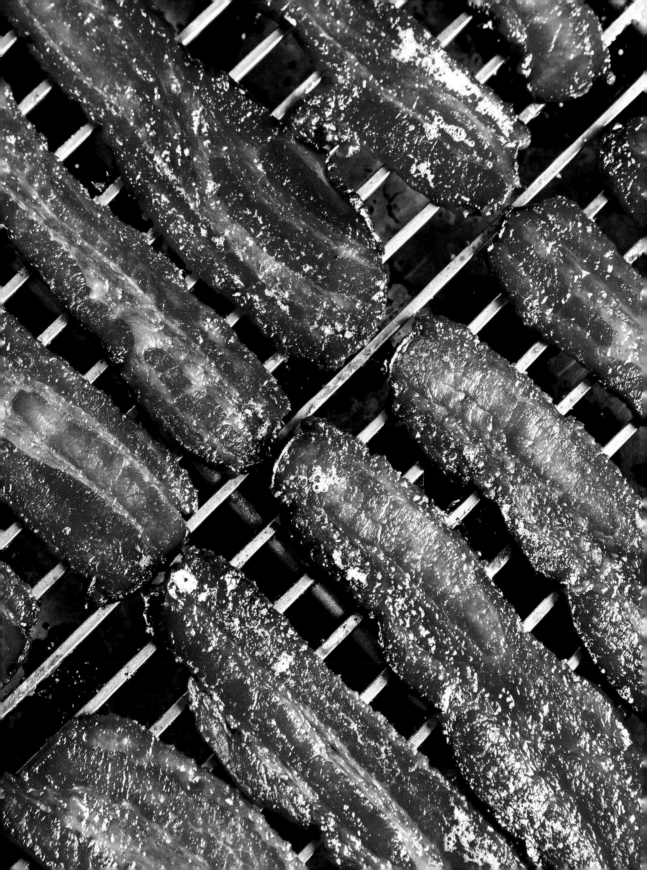

# The Ultimate Breakfast Pan "Cake"

I love the idea of serving my favorite breakfast foods as one giant cake—the ultimate breakfast pancake, to be exact. Layers of scrambled eggs, bacon, and potatoes nestled between pancakes, crowned with whipped cream and fruit, make this breakfast not only fun to eat but also a beautiful and memorable display.

**SERVES 4 TO 6**

**Four cooked 8-inch pancakes**

**1½ cups Roasted Skillet Potatoes (page 39) cut into 1-inch cubes**

**½ pound bacon, cooked**

**1½ cups Perfect Scrambled Eggs (page 36)**

**1 cup lightly sweetened whipped cream**

**1 cup chopped fresh fruit**

**Fresh mint sprigs, for garnish**

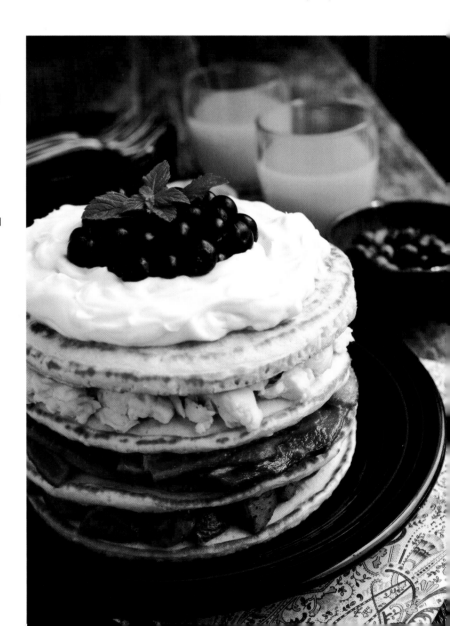

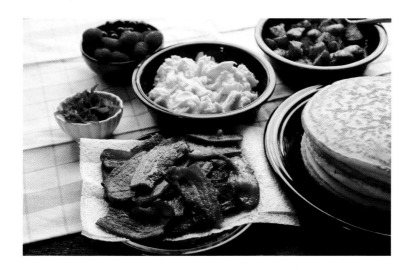

Place a pancake on a plate or serving platter. Add the roasted potatoes, spreading them out to the edge of the pancake. Stack another pancake, followed by a layer of the bacon. Add a third pancake and then a layer of scrambled eggs. Add the final pancake and top it off with the whipped cream, fresh fruit, and mint sprigs.

*Just for fun:* Make mini individual breakfast cakes using waffles for the layers.

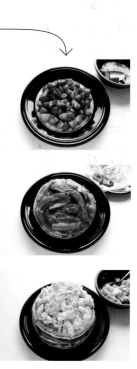

# three

# LUNCH BETWEEN FRIENDS

Having one of my closest friends right down the street has been one of the best perks of living in our neighborhood. I met Alison when she and her husband, Dean, were walking past our house on the way to the park. It was the Fourth of July and Abigail was only six days old. Rob was trimming the laurel hedge outside when I peeked out the window and saw him engaged in conversation with our soon-to-be good friends. As it turns out, Alison had also just given birth to their third child, Myka, a week before Abigail was born. Not only would Myka and Abbi (and eventually Mimi) become the best of friends, but so would Alison and I.

When we spend time together, it usually happens without planning or forethought. This enables us to get together despite our hectic schedules. It's not uncommon for either of us to call the other at any given moment to chat, ask a favor, or suggest a spontaneous walk to the park with the kids. If I need to borrow a cup of flour, I call Alison. If she needs me to pick her kids up from school, I'm there. We have the kind of special relationship that does not hesitate to lend a hand at a moment's notice. There's also a mutual understanding that when we are at each other's house we are there to spend time with one another—turning a blind eye to any piles of clutter that would have otherwise been a deal breaker for having someone over.

There's no pressure to impress Alison with my cooking. Instead, I do my best to pull something together that will not only nourish us physically but also elevate the "kid food" we normally eat on any given day. "If we can't go out to a restaurant for lunch," I say, "bring the restaurant to us." For the short time we're together, we relax in each other's company as our youngest two play. It's friends like Alison who make life meaningful.

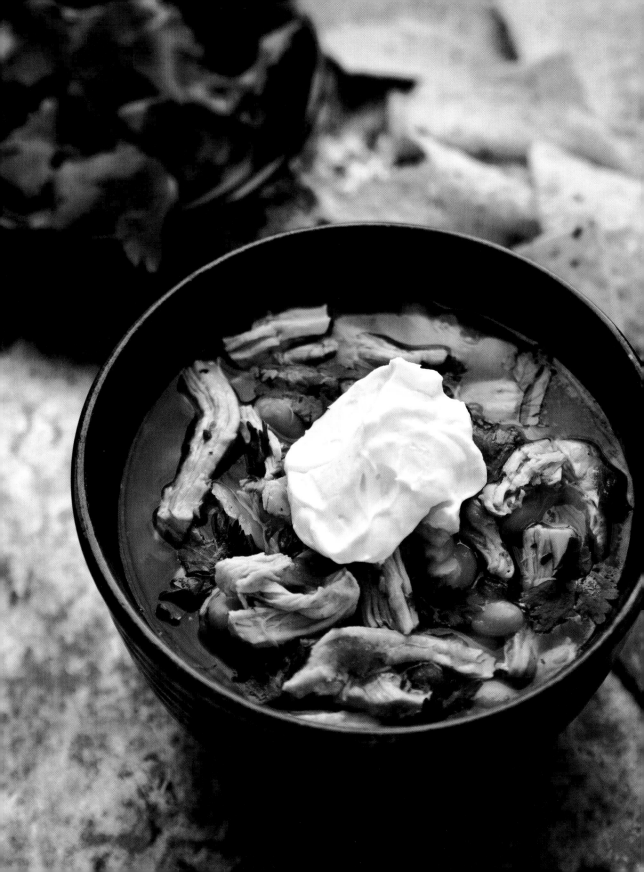

# White Chicken Chili

*Mmmmmm*—this is what Rob always says when eating this chili. With the help of store-bought rotisserie chicken, this soup is full of flavor and can be ready in under 30 minutes. To appreciate this dish in all its glory, be sure not to skip out on the sour cream, cilantro, and a small handful of tortilla chips on the side to really make this chili stand out.

1. In a medium bowl, mix the onion, garlic, jalapeño, cumin, oregano, chili powder, and salt.

2. Heat the olive oil in a large soup pot or Dutch oven over medium heat. Add the onion mixture and cook, stirring occasionally, until the onion has softened, 5 minutes. Pour in the chicken broth and add the bouillon cubes, and bring to a boil. Add the chicken, beans, and green chiles. Cover the pot, reduce the heat, and simmer for 15 minutes to bring the flavors together.

3. To serve, spoon a dollop of sour cream over each bowl of chili and top with about a tablespoon of chopped cilantro. Serve with a side of tortilla chips.

*Cook's note:* This soup has a little kick (heat) to it from the jalapeño, which some children (and adults) may find too spicy. Feel free to use less jalapeño or omit it altogether.

*Time-saving tip:* I like to chop my onions, garlic, and jalapeño all at once in a food processor.

**SERVES 6 TO 8**

1 medium onion, finely chopped

3 garlic cloves, minced

1 jalapeño pepper, seeded and minced

2 teaspoons ground cumin

1 teaspoon dried oregano

½ teaspoon chili powder

½ teaspoon kosher salt

2 tablespoons extra-virgin olive oil

Two 14.5-ounce cans chicken broth

2 chicken bouillon cubes

3 cups chopped rotisserie chicken meat

Two 15-ounce cans cannellini beans or other white beans, drained and rinsed

One 4-ounce can chopped green chiles

½ cup sour cream

½ cup chopped fresh cilantro leaves

Tortilla chips

# Strawberry Spinach Salad

I could eat bowls and bowls of this salad without ever getting tired of it. The sweet, tangy dressing tossed with strawberries makes it a family favorite. It's a classic and vibrant dish to serve at brunches, showers, potlucks, and parties.

**SERVES 4 TO 6**

½ cup distilled white vinegar

½ cup extra-virgin olive oil

⅓ cup honey

2 tablespoons chopped yellow onion

2 tablespoons poppy seeds

½ teaspoon paprika

Two 6-ounce bags fresh baby spinach, washed, dried, and torn into pieces

2 cups sliced fresh strawberries

2 tablespoons toasted sesame seeds

⅓ cup blanched slivered almonds

Add the vinegar, olive oil, honey, onion, poppy seeds, and paprika to a blender and blend until well combined. Pour this dressing over the spinach in a large bowl. Add the strawberries and sesame seeds, and toss to coat lightly but thoroughly. Sprinkle with the almonds. Serve immediately.

*Just for fun:* Add ½ cup crumbled cooked bacon and crumbled goat cheese.

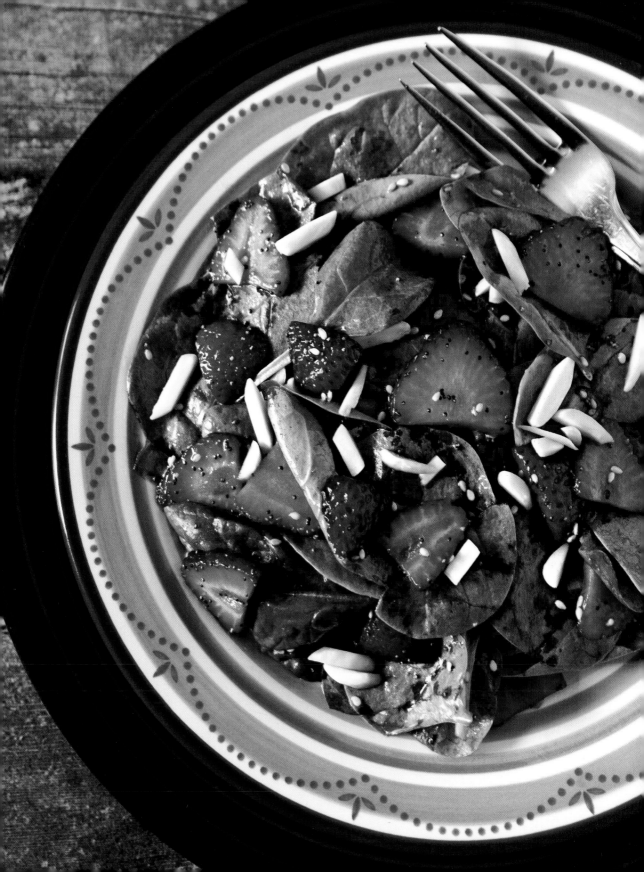

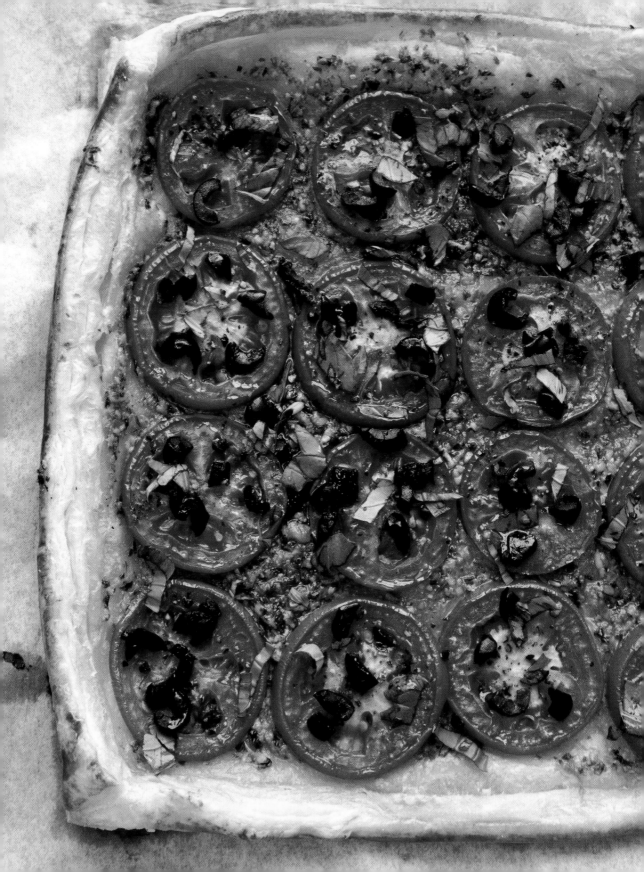

# Tomato Pesto Olive Tart

There's something special about puff pastry that makes everything taste better—especially in this tart. I've always loved the combination of oven-roasted ripe tomatoes with a touch of pesto. Add the bold flavor of Kalamata olives and you have an elegant appetizer for your next party, or a delicious meal for two.

1. Preheat the oven to 400°F. Line a baking sheet with parchment paper.

2. Unfold and roll the puff pastry sheet into a 12-inch square on top of the baking sheet. Make a rim by folding the edges of the pastry square in ½ inch and pressing them down gently. Using a fork, poke holes all over the pastry.

3. Spread the pesto evenly over the pastry (avoiding the rim), using a pastry brush or the back of a spoon. Arrange the tomato slices in a single layer over the entire square, within the rim. Season the tomatoes lightly with salt and pepper, and sprinkle the chopped olives over them.

4. Bake for 20 to 25 minutes, or until the pastry is golden brown. Sprinkle with the basil before serving.

*Just for fun:* Add thinly sliced mozzarella cheese on top of the olives for more of a pizza taste.

**SERVES 6 TO 8 AS AN APPETIZER**

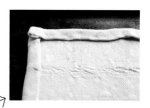

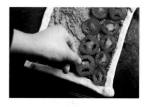

1 sheet frozen puff pastry, thawed

¼ cup Basil Pesto (page 140)

3 ripe Roma tomatoes, sliced ¼ inch thick

Salt and freshly ground pepper

¼ cup chopped Kalamata olives

2 tablespoons chopped fresh basil

# Crab Lemon Basil Pasta

If you've never had pasta tossed in lemon, garlic, and basil, you're in for a real treat. Add ripe cherry tomatoes off the vine and a handful of fresh crabmeat, and you have a simple, fresh, elegant meal the whole family will love.

**SERVES 4**

1 pound spaghetti

⅓ cup extra-virgin olive oil

2 tablespoons unsalted butter

6 to 8 garlic cloves, chopped

1 cup halved cherry tomatoes

½ cup chopped fresh basil

Pinch of kosher salt

Pinch of freshly ground black pepper

½ pound cooked fresh crabmeat

1 lemon, quartered

1. In a large pot, cook the spaghetti in boiling salted water according to the package directions until al dente (tender but firm). Drain the pasta and set aside.

2. Add the olive oil and butter to the same pot and set it over medium heat. When the butter is melted, add the garlic and cook for 30 seconds. Turn off the heat and return the spaghetti to the pot, tossing until it is coated with the garlic sauce. Add the tomatoes, basil, salt, and pepper, and toss gently.

3. Divide the pasta among 4 plates and top each serving with some of the crabmeat. Squeeze 1 lemon quarter over each dish.

*Variation:* Cooked salad shrimp or whole cooked crab cakes can be substituted for the fresh crabmeat. Canned crabmeat is not recommended.

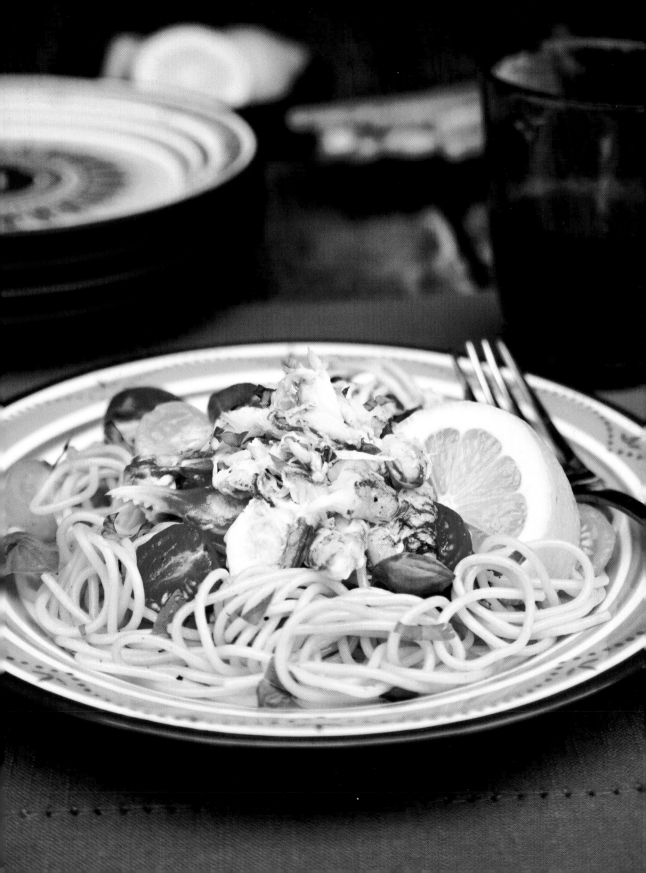

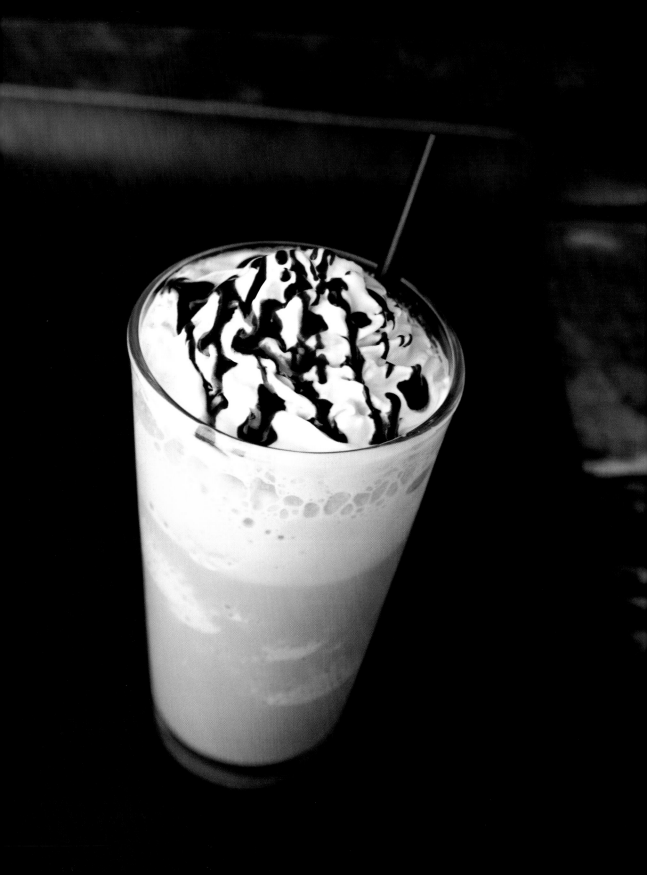

# Coffee Frappe

You know you're in Starbucks country when you live within a three-minute drive of five Starbucks. I cannot drive in any direction without passing the green mermaid, tempting me to spend $5 on an afternoon Frappuccino. Save yourself some coin for a special night out and make your own at home.

Combine the ice, coffee, milk, and sugar in a blender, and puree for 30 to 45 seconds. Pour the frappe into a tall glass. Top it off with whipped cream and drizzle with chocolate syrup.

*Variation:* For a mocha frappe, reduce the sugar to 2 tablespoons and add 2 tablespoons of chocolate syrup when blending.

**SERVES 1**

1¼ cups ice cubes

¾ cup extra-strong brewed coffee

½ cup milk (any kind)

3 tablespoons granulated sugar

Whipped cream (fresh or from a canister)

Chocolate syrup

# four

# TWEEN BIRTHDAY BASH

When my daughter Abigail turned ten years old, it was a big deal—she was now counting the years in double digits. What happened to the little girl who used to live in Disney princess dresses, clutching her favorite teddy bear as she fell asleep in her daddy's arms? Suddenly our little girl wasn't so little.

Planning her own birthday party was of great importance to Abigail, and I was so proud of her for taking the initiative. She took great pride in making her own invitations and delegating tasks to Rob and me. My job was catering.

At ten Abigail was beyond serving Goldfish crackers. She handed me a list of menu items she wanted me to make:

- Coconut Chicken Tenders
- Caramel Corn
- Fruit Salsa with Baked Cinnamon Chips
- Peaches 'n' Cream Italian Cream Sodas
- Vanilla Birthday Cake with Buttercream Frosting
- Chocolate Cookies 'n' Cream Ice Cream

I remembered when I could get away with serving dinosaur-shaped chicken nuggets, apple slices, popcorn, and juice boxes! Now that Abigail was older, she wanted the food to reflect her personal style without interference from me. I don't blame her. I remember feeling pretty grown up when I was ten too.

After an evening of loud dance music, games, eating, singing "Happy Birthday," and opening presents, I walked over to the couch, sat down, and lifted my feet to the coffee table. With my eyes closed, I felt Abigail's arms wrap around me as we cuddled and recalled every fun detail of a birthday well celebrated. I reminded her that while she may be ten years old, she would always be my baby, and resting her head on my shoulder, she told me she wished she could stay ten forever. I quietly responded, "I wish that too." As she fell sleep, I reminded myself that as tired as I was, there were only a few birthdays left where she'd let me be as involved as I was for this party. And with that, I surrendered to my exhausted body and fell asleep too.

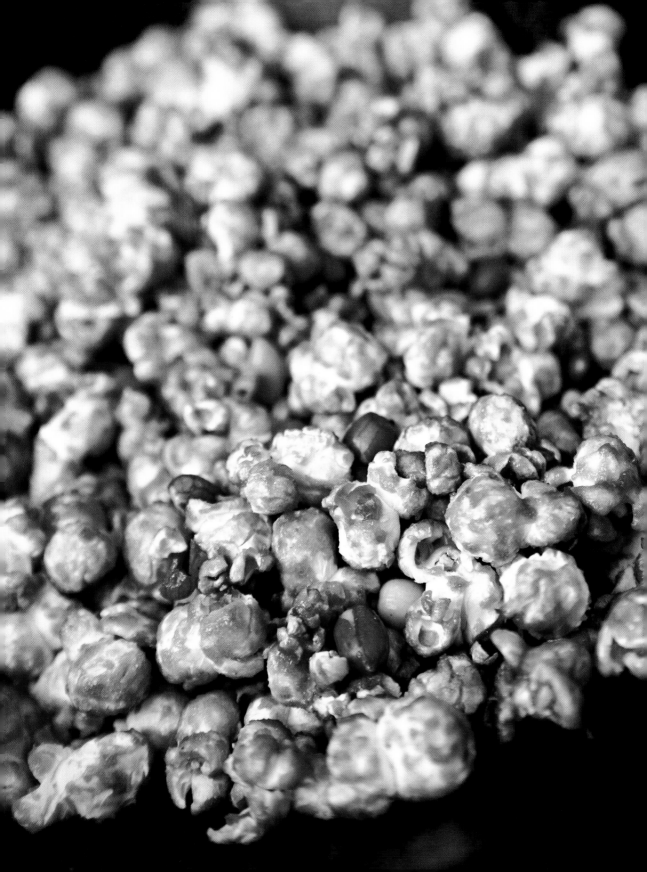

# Caramel Corn

The candy caramel coating combined with a hint of salt makes this savory, sweet snack addictive. I usually make large batches of this beloved treat for parties and kids' sleepovers. It is always a hit with every age group. There's never a piece left in the bowl.

1. Preheat the oven to 300°F. Spray 2 baking sheets with nonstick cooking spray and set aside.

2. Pop the popcorn in an air popper or in a large, heavy covered pot over low heat. Place the popcorn and the peanuts in a clean paper grocery bag.

3. In a medium saucepan over medium-high heat, combine the brown sugar, corn syrup, butter, and 1 teaspoon of the salt. Bring to a boil and cook for 5 minutes, stirring occasionally. Turn off the heat and stir in the vanilla and baking soda. Pour this caramel sauce into the grocery bag and stir the sauce, popcorn, and nuts with a wooden spoon until the popcorn is coated.

4. Spread the popcorn evenly over the 2 baking sheets. Sprinkle 1½ teaspoons of the remaining salt over each batch. Bake for 45 minutes, stirring the popcorn every 15 minutes. Allow the caramel corn to cool before serving. Store any leftovers in zip-top bags or in an airtight container.

*Lighter note:* Cut the caramel sauce ingredients in half for a less sweet caramel corn.

**MAKES 16 CUPS**

½ cup unpopped popcorn kernels

One 12-ounce can Spanish peanuts

1½ cups firmly packed dark brown sugar

⅓ cup light corn syrup

8 tablespoons (1 stick) unsalted butter

4 teaspoons kosher salt

½ teaspoon pure vanilla extract

½ teaspoon baking soda

# Fruit Salsa with Baked Cinnamon Chips

I love traditional salsa and tortilla chips for a savory snack, but this fruit salsa with cinnamon chips is a fun sweet alternative. Adding basil to the fruit may seem strange, but it actually complements the sweetness of the fruit and the cinnamon in the chips. It's just one of those things you have to try to believe it!

**MAKES 4 CUPS**

FRUIT SALSA

**Juice of 1 lime**

**2 tablespoons granulated sugar**

**½ teaspoon ground cinnamon**

**4 fresh basil leaves, chopped**

**1 kiwi, peeled and cut into ¼-inch dice**

**1 crisp apple, peeled, cored, and cut into ¼-inch dice**

**1 cup strawberries, hulled and cut into ¼-inch dice**

**1 mango, peeled, pitted, and cut into ¼-inch dice**

BAKED CINNAMON CHIPS

**Eight 10-inch flour tortillas**

**Butter-flavored cooking spray**

**1 cup cinnamon sugar (scant 1 cup granulated sugar plus 2 tablespoons ground cinnamon)**

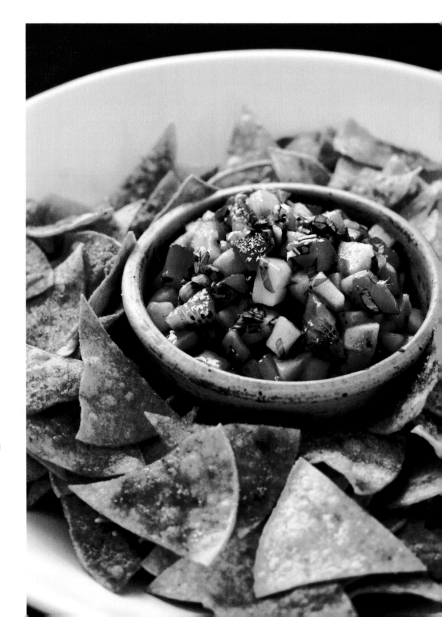

1. To make the fruit salsa, whisk the lime juice, sugar, cinnamon, and basil together in a small bowl. In a large bowl, combine the kiwi, apple, strawberries, and mango. Pour the lime juice mixture over the fruit and mix gently. Transfer to a large serving bowl.

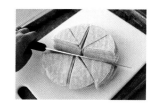

2. To make the cinnamon chips, preheat the oven to 350°F.

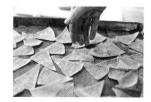

3. Coat each side of the tortillas with cooking spray. Make a single stack of the tortillas and slice through the stack to make 8 wedges from each tortilla. Working in batches, spread the tortilla wedges in a single layer on a large baking sheet. Sprinkle the wedges with cinnamon sugar, and spray them again with cooking spray. Bake for 8 to 10 minutes, until nice and crispy. Repeat to make the rest of the cinnamon chips. Allow the chips to cool for 15 minutes before serving.

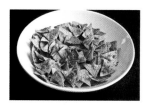

*Make-ahead tip:* Store the chopped fruit in separate containers in the refrigerator until ready to serve. Prep the dressing and store until ready to use. Toss the salsa ingredients together right before serving.

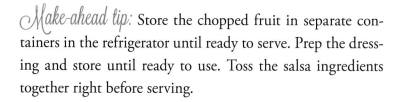

# Coconut Chicken Tenders

These chicken tenders are a hit with my family. Crusted with sweetened coconut and panko breadcrumbs, these flavorful chicken strips disappear quickly in our home. They're the number one most requested dinner item.

**SERVES 4 TO 6**

Peanut, canola, or vegetable oil, for frying

2 pounds chicken breast tenderloins

Kosher salt and freshly ground black pepper

½ cup orange juice

½ cup sweetened condensed milk

1 egg, beaten

1½ cups panko breadcrumbs

1 cup shredded sweetened coconut

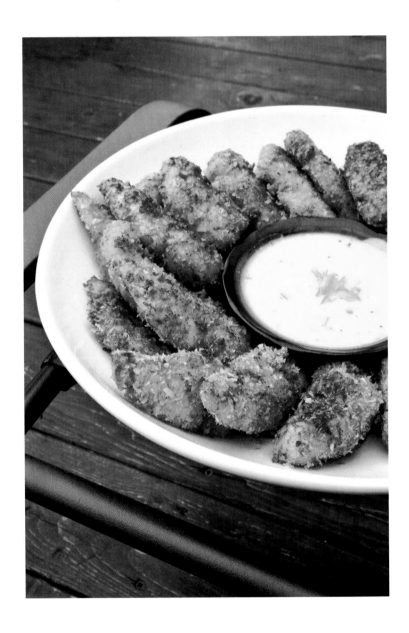

1. Heat 3 inches of peanut oil in a large heavy-duty pot or a deep-fryer to 350°F or medium heat.

2. Spread the chicken tenders out on a cookie sheet and season them with salt and pepper on both sides. Set aside.

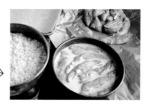

3. In a medium bowl, mix the orange juice, condensed milk, and egg until well combined. In a medium shallow dish, combine the panko crumbs and coconut.

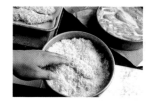

4. Coat each chicken tender in the wet mixture, then in the panko-coconut mixture. Set aside.

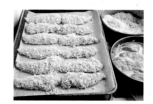

5. Fry the chicken tenders for 3 to 4 minutes on each side, or until golden brown. Transfer the cooked chicken to a plate lined with a paper towel to soak up any excess oil. Remove the paper towel before serving.

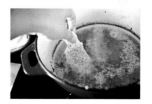

*Just for fun:* Use crushed cornflakes instead of the panko.

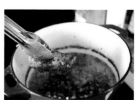

# Chocolate Cookies 'n' Cream Dairy-Free "Ice Cream"

This is the best four-ingredient ice cream you will ever eat. Made with coconut milk, cocoa powder, sugar, and crushed Oreo cookies, it's so silky and creamy that you'd never guess it is dairy-free. I developed this recipe for Abigail, who is sensitive to dairy, so she could enjoy her favorite ice cream flavor without suffering the consequences later. The result is so amazing that it's become one of my favorite "ice creams" too!

**MAKES 1 PINT**

One 14-ounce can coconut milk

⅓ cup granulated sugar

2 tablespoons unsweetened cocoa powder

10 Oreos, crushed

Combine the coconut milk, sugar, and cocoa powder in a blender and blend for 20 seconds. Pour the liquid into the bowl of an ice cream maker and churn according to the manufacturer's directions. In the last 5 minutes of churning, add the crushed Oreos. Transfer the ice cream to a plastic container, cover, and store in the freezer until ready to eat.

*Note:* Chaokoh brand coconut milk works best with this recipe because of its high fat content.

*Just for fun:* For mocha cookies 'n' cream ice cream, add a shot of cooled brewed espresso to the liquid mixture before churning it.

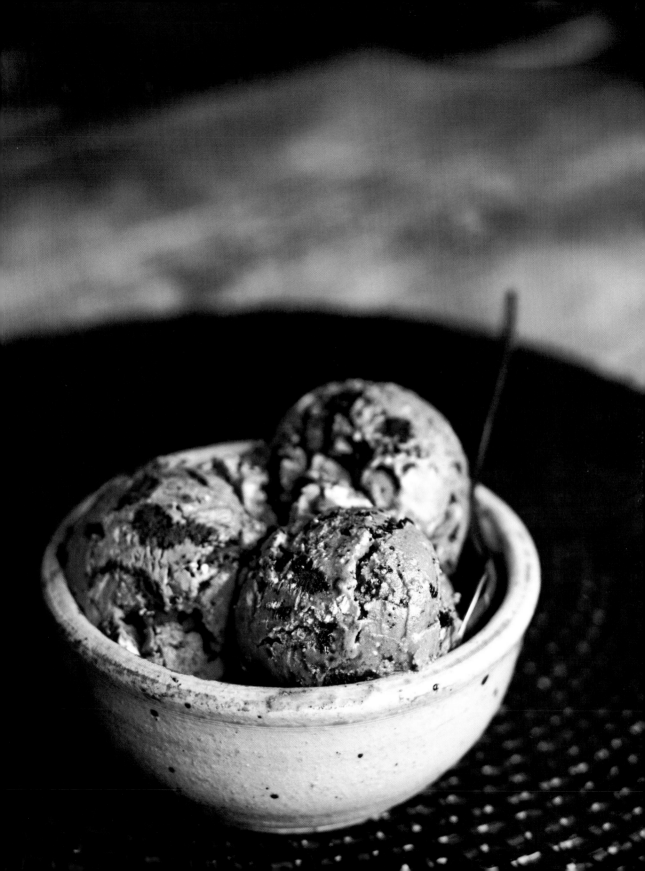

# Peaches 'n' Cream Italian Cream Soda

When I worked at an espresso bar, I would experiment with making different combinations of Italian cream sodas just for fun. One of my favorite flavors is the combination of peach and vanilla. The sweet fruit is balanced by the vanilla, making this a popular party drink for all ages.

**SERVES 1**

Ice cubes

1 cup club soda or sparkling water

3 tablespoons peach-flavored syrup

1 tablespoon vanilla-flavored syrup

2 tablespoons half-and-half

Fill a tall glass with ice. Pour in the club soda, followed by the peach and vanilla syrups. Top the drink off with the half-and-half, and serve it with a straw for people to mix it up themselves.

*Where to buy flavored syrups:* Flavored syrups can be found in the coffee section of many grocery stores. Common brands include Torani and DaVinci.

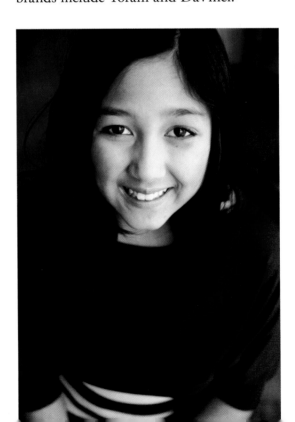

# All-Occasion Vanilla Cake with Buttercream Frosting and Sour Cream Raspberry Filling

Good-bye cake mix, good-bye supermarket bakery, and hello scratch baking! Nothing beats a homemade cake baked with love, especially when it's a birthday cake. Once you go scratch, you'll never go back!

1. Preheat the oven to 350°F. Generously grease two 9-inch cake pans with nonstick cooking spray. Line the cake pans with parchment paper by cutting paper rounds to fit the bottom of each pan.

2. Using an electric hand or stand mixer, cream the butter, oil, and sugar together on medium speed for 3 minutes, until light and fluffy. Add the eggs and egg yolks one at a time, waiting for each egg to be mixed in before adding another. Add the vanilla, baking powder, and salt. Pour in the flour and milk, and mix for 2 minutes, until the batter is smooth. Scrape the sides and bottom of the bowl with a rubber spatula and mix for 1 minute more.

3. Pour the cake batter evenly into the 2 cake pans. Using both hands, grab the sides of each cake pan and gently tap the bottom of the pan on the kitchen counter a few times. (This helps burst any air bubbles trapped in the batter, allowing for a tight crumb texture.)

**MAKES A TWO-LAYER 9-INCH CAKE**

1 cup (2 sticks) unsalted butter, at room temperature

⅓ cup vegetable oil

2¼ cups granulated sugar

3 eggs

3 egg yolks

1 tablespoon pure vanilla extract

1 tablespoon baking powder

½ teaspoon salt

3 cups cake flour

1 cup whole milk

Classic American Buttercream Frosting (recipe follows)

Whipped Sour Cream Filling with Fresh Raspberries (recipe follows)

**4.** Bake for 35 to 40 minutes, until the center of the cakes spring back when touched (or see the testing method below). Allow the cake layers to cool in their pans for 15 minutes.

**5.** To release each cake from its pan, slowly and carefully run a butter knife along the side of the pan. Then grab each side of the cake pan and gently shake it up and down and side to side to loosen the cake before inverting it onto a wire rack to cool. Allow the cake layers to cool completely.

**6.** Following the instructions on page 73, place one cooled cake layer on a serving platter cut side up, or better yet on a cake round, and pipe a rim of the buttercream frosting. Spread the sour cream filling over the layer within the rim, and dot it with the raspberries, pressing them gently into the filling. Place the second cake layer on top, bottom side up, and then frost the top and sides of the cake with the buttercream.

*Testing the cake for doneness:* Stick a wooden skewer into the center of a cake layer and remove it quickly. If the stick is clean of any cake batter, with only a few crumbs, the cake is completely baked. If any batter comes up, bake the cake for 5 minutes longer and test again.

*Avoiding disaster:* Do not let the cake layers cool in the pans for longer than 15 minutes after removing them from the oven. Otherwise they will adhere to the pans.

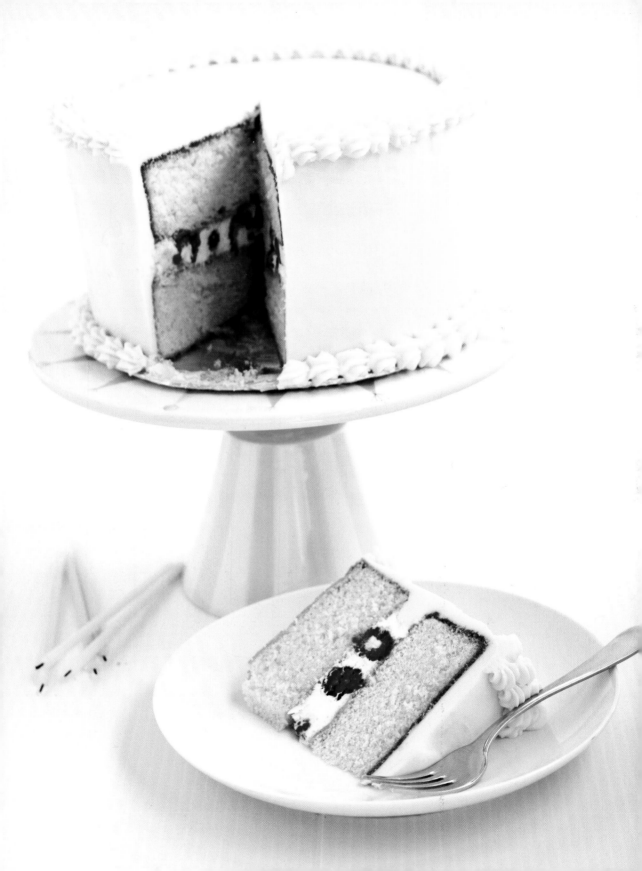

# Whipped Sour Cream Filling with Fresh Raspberries

Cake fillings may be sandwiched between layers of cake, but that doesn't mean they should play second fiddle to the frosting. A good filling can elevate the satisfaction level with every bite. One of my favorite fillings pairs fresh fruit with sweetened whipped cream. Add a little sour cream for some extra zing and you have the perfect filling for a memorable cake.

**MAKES 2½ CUPS**

½ cup heavy cream

¼ teaspoon pure vanilla extract

½ cup confectioners' sugar, sifted

½ cup sour cream

1 cup fresh raspberries

1. Using a hand or stand mixer, whip the heavy cream and vanilla extract together on medium-high speed until stiff peaks form. Turn the mixer off and add the confectioners' sugar and sour cream. Turn the mixer back on at the lowest speed and whip for 1 minute. Then increase the speed to medium and whip for 1 minute more.

2. Spread the filling on top of each layer of cake as called for in the recipe, and dot the raspberries over the filling. Gently press the raspberries down before stacking the next layer of cake. (This filling can also be used as a frosting on single-layer cakes.) The filling will keep for up to a week, refrigerated.

*Just for fun:* Use the Whipped Sour Cream Filling as a fruit dip or as a topping on pancakes, shortcakes, waffles, French toast, pies, and ice cream.

# Classic American Buttercream Frosting

It's very sad when bad frosting happens to good cake. You know, when someone goes out of their way to bake a homemade cake only to use canned frosting or a frosting made with shortening, leaving a greasy aftertaste in your mouth—gross. This buttercream frosting is made of pure butter whipped to the perfect consistency for all your frosting and decorating needs.

**MAKES 4 TO 4½ CUPS**

**1 pound unsalted butter, slightly cooler than room temperature**

**5 to 6 cups confectioners' sugar, sifted**

**1 tablespoon pure vanilla extract, or 1½ teaspoons almond extract**

**½ teaspoon salt**

**¼ to ½ cup heavy cream or whole milk**

Using an electric hand or stand mixer, cream the butter for 1 minute on medium speed. Turn the mixer off and add 5 cups of the confectioners' sugar. Turn the mixer back on at the lowest speed (so the sugar doesn't blow everywhere). Once all the sugar has been incorporated into the butter, increase the mixer speed to medium and add the vanilla, salt, and ¼ cup of the cream. Beat for 3 minutes. If you prefer a frosting with a stiff consistency, add the remaining cup of confectioners' sugar. If your frosting needs to be thinned out, add the remaining cream, 1 tablespoon at a time. Use immediately or store in a sealed container in the refrigerator for up to 1 month.

*Variations:* Feel free to substitute different flavored extracts, including lemon and coconut. For chocolate buttercream, add ¼ cup unsweetened cocoa powder. Adding lemon zest or a little orange juice concentrate will also enhance the flavor in a delightful way.

# How to Frost a Cake

Homemade cakes should be as beautiful on the outside as they are tasty on the inside. If the idea of frosting a layered cake has ever intimidated you, this step-by-step visual tutorial will help you conquer your fear and transform you into an expert cake decorator.

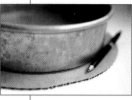

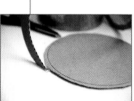

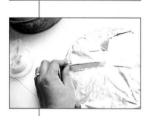

### Step 1—Making a covered cake board

A covered cake board will give your cake a more polished look. Cake boards are easy to make if you have a large pastry board or a piece of thick cardboard. Center the cake pan on top of a piece of cardboard and trace a line around the pan. Cut the cardboard ½ inch wider than the traced line. Place the board on top of a larger piece of aluminum foil and fold the foil tightly over the board, securing the edges with tape. Turn the board over and use the foil-covered side as the "viewable" side.

**What you'll need:**

Cake board/cardboard

Aluminum foil

Tape

4 cups frosting, such as the buttercream opposite (I do not recommend canned frosting)

Two 8- or 9-inch baked cake layers

1 cup cake filling, such as the Whipped Sour Cream Filling (page 71)

Offset spatula

Pastry bag or 2 zip-top bags

Cake turntable or lazy Susan
(If you don't have one, don't worry. Having a turntable makes it easier to frost but isn't necessary.)

### Step 2—Adhering the cake to the board

If you prefer the top of your cake layers to be level and flat, first trim away the "dome" of each cake by taking a bread knife and carefully slicing it off.

Spread a few tablespoons of frosting on the center of the viewable side of the cake board. (This will function as a "glue" to adhere the cake to the board.) Place one of the cake layers on top of the board, keeping it as centered as possible. Gently press the cake down so that it sticks to the frosting. Set the cake on a turntable. (If you don't have one, you can use a flat-bottomed mixing bowl that is slightly smaller than the cake board. Place a towel over the bowl, and then set the board with the cake on top of the bowl. Be sure the cake is centered over the bowl, and take care when turning the cake.)

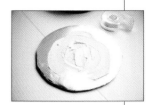

### Step 3—Filling the cake

Fill a pastry bag with a large circle tip or a zip-top bag with frosting. (If you're using a zip-top bag, cut ½ inch off a bottom corner of the bag.) Twist the top of the bag a few times to keep the frosting from leaking out. Hold the bag in your hand, securing the cinched part of the bag with your thumb and pointer finger. Apply enough pressure to the bag so the frosting starts to pipe out from the tip. Pipe a ½-inch edge around the perimeter of the top of the cake layer. This is called a "dam." There are two reasons for creating a dam: First, it holds the filling inside the cake and keeps it from oozing out and mixing with the frosting. Second, it helps patch and fill in any uneven spots around the cake.

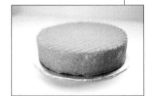

Now spread your choice of filling inside the dam. The filling should reach no higher than the top of the dam.

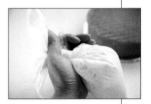

Once the cake is filled, set the top layer, bottom side up, over the bottom layer, centering it carefully. Gently press the top layer down for the filling to adhere to it. Pipe more frosting between the cake layers. This will help fill any gaps for a more seamless look.

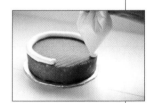

### Step 4—Making the crumb coating

Using the back side of an offset spatula, smooth out any frosting that may have oozed out between the layers of cake, rotating the cake as you go.

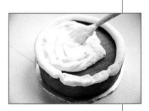

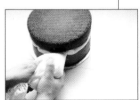

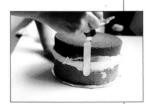

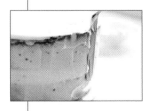

Brush off any excess crumbs with a pastry brush or by gently rubbing the palm of your hand around the cake.

Spoon about 1 cup of frosting on top of the cake. Starting with the top of the cake and working your way around the sides, spread a thin layer of frosting over the entire cake.

This crumb coating serves two purposes: First, it will trap those pesky crumbs and keep them from being mixed in with the outer layer of frosting. Second, it works as a primer or base for a second layer of frosting, filling in any imperfections in the cake. Using an offset spatula, smooth out the frosting as best as you can. Don't worry if the frosting is transparent enough to see the cake beneath it.

Chill your cake in the refrigerator for 30 minutes to 1 hour to allow it to set up. This will make it easy to apply another coat of frosting.

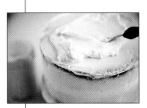

### Step 5—Frosting the cake

Remove the cake from the refrigerator. Gently touch the cake. If no frosting pulls up, your cake is ready for its final coat. If any frosting sticks to your finger, refrigerate the cake for another 15 minutes.

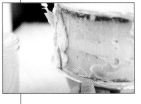

Place about 2 cups of frosting on top of the cake. Start icing the cake, working from the top down and around the sides. Add more frosting as needed.

For clean edges on top, take the edge of your spatula and drag it toward the center of your cake. Do this around the perimeter of your cake. For a smooth finish, use the back side of your spatula in one direction, sweeping across the cake from edge to edge and all around the sides, rotating the cake as you go.

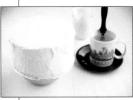

If you want to smooth the cake out even more, fill a tall mug with boiling water. Allow the spatula to warm up in the hot water for 30 seconds. Grab the spatula and quickly wipe off any water with a paper towel. Continue to smooth the frosting as you did before; you'll notice that the warmth of the spatula

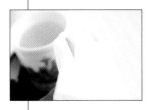

melts the seams of the frosting for a more flawless finish. Feel free to reheat the spatula in the hot water and continue to smooth out the frosting until you are happy with how smooth your cake is.

Taking a damp paper towel, wipe the exposed edge of the cake board to clean off any excess frosting.

Voilà, you did it!

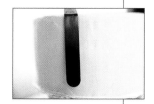

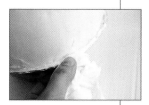

### Just for fun—piping borders

Adding a decorative border around the base and top edge of the cake is a great finishing touch to complete your masterpiece. Fill a zip-top bag with a cup of frosting and snip off ¼ inch from a bottom corner. Twist the top of the bag a few times to keep the frosting from leaking out. Hold the bag in your hand, securing the cinched part of the bag with your thumb and pointer finger. Apply enough pressure to the bag so that the frosting starts to pipe out from the corner. Holding the bag at a 45-degree angle, slowly apply enough pressure at the base of the cake for a bead of frosting the size of a pea to come out. Release the pressure and pull the bag away for a sideways teardrop to form. Starting at the tail of the teardrop, repeat, piping more teardrops around the cake to form a border. This same technique can be used to pipe a decorative edge on top of the cake as well. For a pearl effect, pipe small beads without a tail.

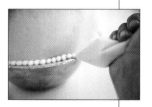

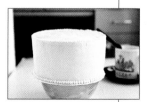

# five

# FATHER'S DAY

From the moment our first daughter was born, my husband, Rob, was a transformed man and quickly became one of the most involved dads I've ever known. When he's not at work, you can find him volunteering at school, playing soccer with the kids outside, and taking special weekend trips involving camping, snowboarding, golfing, and other dad-centric adventures. He's the best dad a kid could ever hope for, and I'm eternally grateful for the way he loves our kids.

Every Father's Day, the kids and I try to make the whole day as special as we can. Part of our annual tradition is to let him sleep in as long as he wants to, bringing him breakfast in bed when he shows signs of waking up. I don't know anyone who appreciates having a hot cup of coffee delivered to him more than Rob does.

Sitting around him on the bed, the kids wait eagerly for him to finish breakfast so each of them can hand him their homemade cards and gifts. "Daddy, me first! Open mine first!" one will say. The other kids follow with similar pleas. He opens each card with tears of happiness in his eyes.

The rest of our day is spent being together as a family while I cook his favorite Asian-inspired dishes. At the end of the evening, he tucks the kids into their beds. Each year I can hear Rob telling them, "This has been the best Father's Day ever." He gives each of them one last kiss and hug for the night and joins me on the couch to soak in the day. He is one proud papa, and it shows.

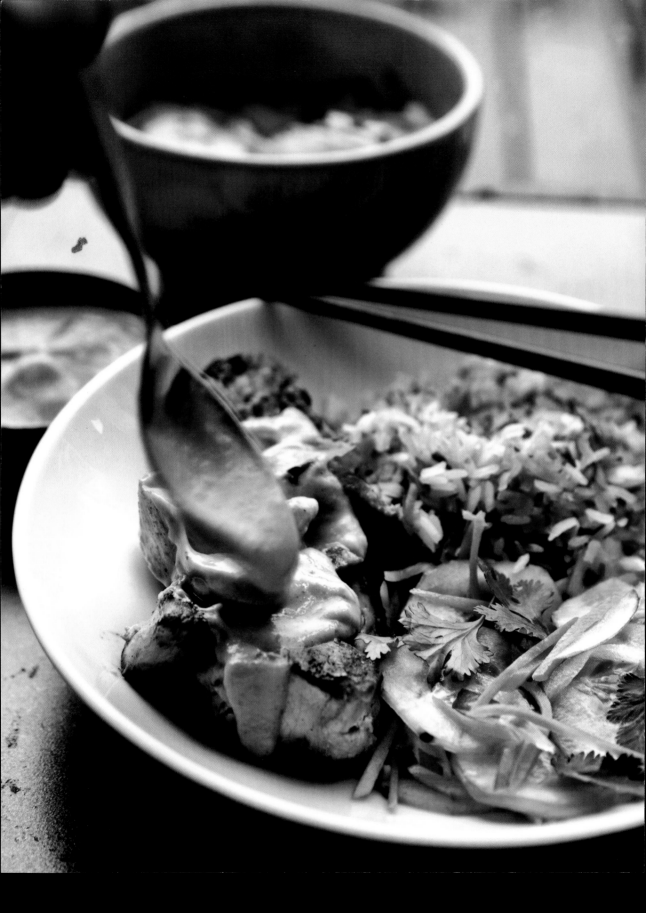

# Asian Cucumber Salad

I love the refreshing sweet and tangy flavors of this salad, especially when it's served alongside grilled meat and vegetables. My husband, a cucumber lover, can never get enough of it.

Combine the vinegar, sugar, and salt in a microwave-safe bowl, and heat for 20 seconds in the microwave. Stir until the sugar is completely dissolved. In a small bowl, toss the cucumber, carrot, red onion, and cilantro with the vinegar dressing. Chill in the refrigerator for 30 minutes before serving.

*Cook's note:* This salad is meant to be served as a small side dish with a larger meal.

*Like it spicy?* Add a pinch of red pepper flakes or Asian garlic chili sauce to the salad.

**MAKES 2 CUPS; SERVES 4 AS A SMALL SIDE DISH**

⅓ cup rice vinegar

2 tablespoons granulated sugar

¼ teaspoon salt

1 large cucumber, peeled and thinly sliced

1 carrot, peeled and cut into matchsticks

¼ cup thinly sliced red onion

3 tablespoons chopped fresh cilantro

*Asian Cucumber Salad served with Coconut Rice (page 80) and Thai Marinated Grilled Chicken Skewers (page 86)*

# Coconut Rice

Jasmine rice is an aromatic medium-grain rice traditionally served with Thai food. After being frustrated with countless attempts at making coconut rice using coconut milk, I came up with a simple and flavorful method that makes the best-tasting coconut rice I've ever had. And the best part of it all is that it uses only two ingredients: rice and toasted sweetened coconut!

**SERVES 4 TO 6**

**1 cup shredded sweetened coconut**

**4 cups warm cooked jasmine rice**

Set a large nonstick frying pan over medium heat. Add the coconut and stir frequently until most of the flakes are aromatic, toasted, and browned, 3 to 4 minutes. Immediately transfer the toasted coconut to a large bowl. Add the warm rice to the bowl, and mix the rice and coconut continuously with a rice paddle or wooden spoon for 2 to 3 minutes, until the rice has changed color from white to light brown.

*Just for fun:* Drizzle some Peanut Coconut Sauce (page 88) over the coconut rice. It's a great combination.

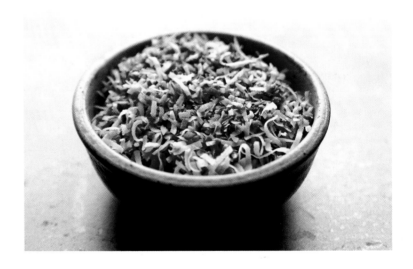

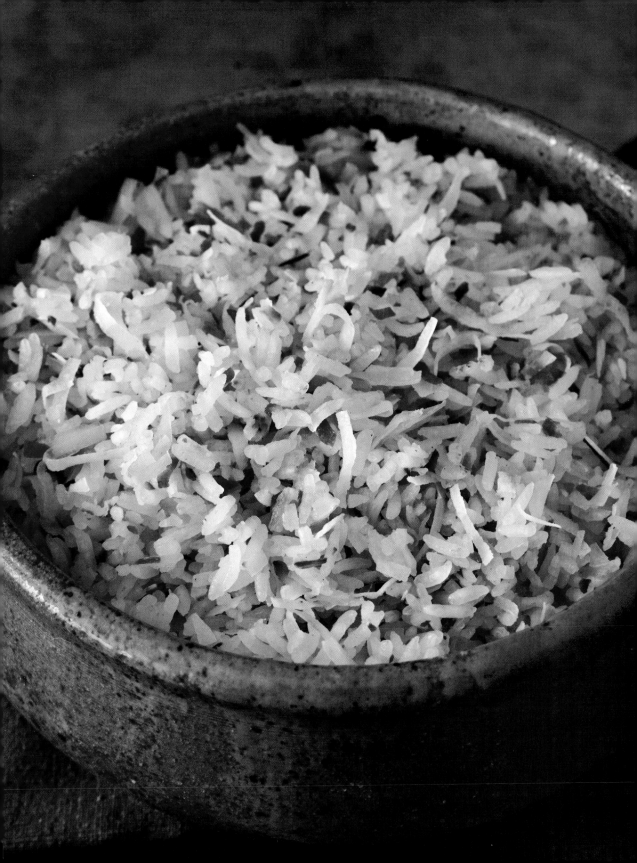

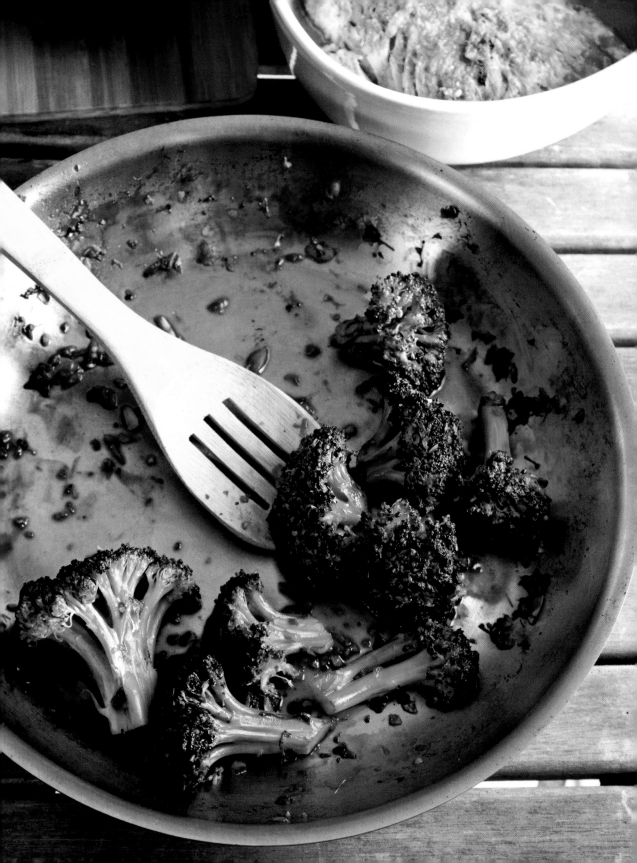

# Stir-Fry Garlic Ginger Broccoli

Broccoli is a staple side dish in our home. One of my very favorite ways to dress it up is to stir-fry the broccoli in a light garlic and ginger sauce. The secret to stir-frying broccoli is to blanch it first, then quickly fry it for a perfectly tender-crisp, Asian-inspired dish.

1. Fill a large bowl with ice water and set it aside.

2. Bring a large pot of salted water to a boil. Drop the broccoli into the boiling water and cook for 2 minutes. Immediately drain the broccoli and transfer it to the bowl of ice water to stop the cooking and to keep the broccoli crisp. Use a slotted spoon to transfer the cooled broccoli from the ice bath to a paper-towel-lined plate to absorb the excess water.

3. Whisk the garlic, ginger, soy sauce, oyster sauce, honey, and 2 tablespoons of water in a small bowl. Heat the olive oil in a large frying pan or wok set over medium heat. When the oil is hot, add the broccoli to the pan and cook for 2 minutes to sear the broccoli, turning every 30 seconds. Add the sauce to the pan. When the sauce begins to bubble, toss the broccoli for 2 minutes with a wooden spoon. Serve immediately.

*Like it spicy?* Stir ½ teaspoon of red pepper flakes into the sauce for added heat.

**SERVES 4 TO 6**

2 broccoli crowns, cut into florets

8 garlic cloves, minced

2 tablespoons minced fresh ginger

2 tablespoons soy sauce

2 tablespoons oyster sauce

2 tablespoons honey

2 tablespoons extra-virgin olive oil or vegetable oil

# Sesame Ginger King Salmon Fillets

Living in the Pacific Northwest has its privileges, fresh salmon being one of them. My favorite type of salmon is the wild king, or Chinook, variety. It's nice and thick, with the least amount of "fishy" taste and smell. When cooked properly, it's the tenderest and most delicious salmon of them all, rightfully earning its name as king of all salmon.

**SERVES 4**

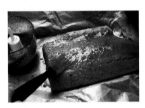

¼ cup plus
2 tablespoons
firmly packed dark
brown sugar

¼ cup Asian sesame oil

3 tablespoons rice vinegar

2 tablespoons soy sauce

1 tablespoon minced fresh ginger

1 garlic clove

4 center-cut king salmon fillets (6 to 8 ounces each)

Kosher salt and freshly ground black pepper

2 tablespoons toasted black sesame seeds

1. Preheat the oven to 450°F. Line a rimmed baking sheet with parchment paper or aluminum foil.

2. To make the sesame ginger sauce, blend the brown sugar, sesame oil, rice vinegar, soy sauce, ginger, and garlic in a food processor or blender until everything is emulsified. Divide the sauce between 2 bowls.

3. Place the salmon fillets, skin side down, on the baking sheet. Season the fillets with salt and pepper. Generously brush each fillet with the sauce from one of the bowls.

4. Bake the fish for 15 minutes, or until opaque (less if you like it a little pink in the middle). Transfer the salmon to serving plates and pour the sauce from the remaining bowl over each fillet. Sprinkle the salmon with the sesame seeds, and serve.

*Leftover salmon?* I love cooking fresh pasta and adding the leftover salmon and sauce to it. Toss it with some cooked broccoli, asparagus, or spinach and you have yourself a great meal.

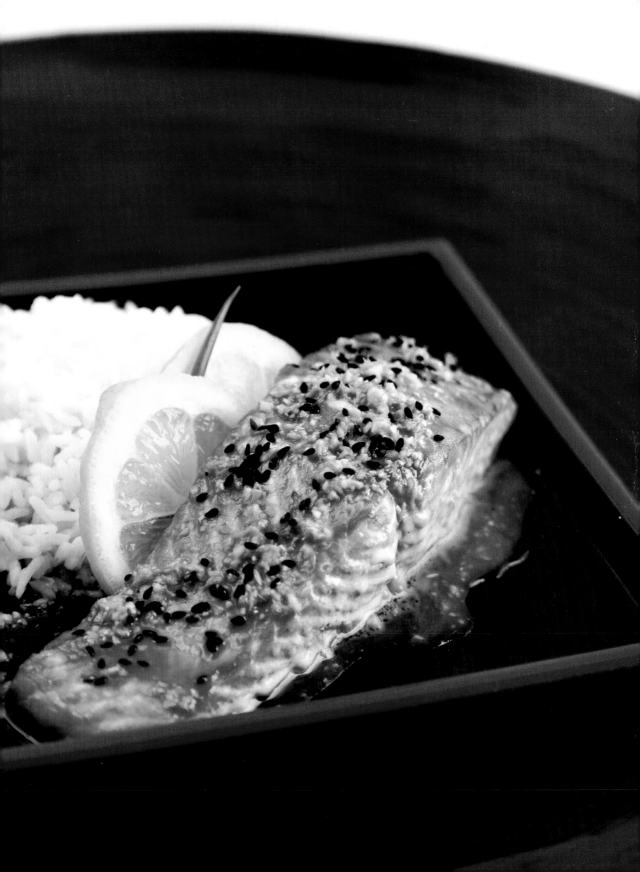

# Thai Marinated Grilled Chicken Skewers

My kids cannot resist these tender, juicy Asian-inspired chicken skewers. The combination of ginger, cardamom, and curry, sweetened by brown sugar, is sweet, savory, and bold! Serve them with a side of peanut coconut sauce and your taste buds will thank you.

**SERVES 4 TO 6**

*Special equipment:*
**24 wooden skewers**

**3 pounds skinless, boneless chicken breasts, cut into 1-inch cubes**

MARINADE

**¼ cup soy sauce**

**3 tablespoons firmly packed dark brown sugar**

**2 tablespoons fresh lime juice**

**2 tablespoons oil**

**1 tablespoon curry powder**

**2 garlic cloves, minced**

**1 teaspoon finely minced fresh ginger**

**½ teaspoon ground cardamom**

**Peanut Coconut Sauce (recipe follows), for serving**

1. Soak the skewers in ice-cold water for 15 minutes to prevent them from burning; then set them aside.

2. Place the chicken in a medium bowl. Whisk all the marinade ingredients together in a separate bowl. Pour the marinade over the chicken and massage the meat with your hands for 1 minute to coat the cubes well. Cover the bowl with plastic wrap and marinate in the refrigerator for at least 1 hour or as long as overnight.

3. Spray a grill rack with nonstick cooking spray and set the heat to high or use a grill pan. Thread 6 to 8 chicken cubes onto each skewer. When the grill is ready, cook the chicken for 8 to 10 minutes, turning the skewers over halfway through. Remove the skewers from the grill and allow the chicken to rest for a few minutes before serving.

4. Serve the Peanut Coconut Sauce alongside.

*Variations:* Cubes of top sirloin beef or pork loin can be substituted for the chicken.

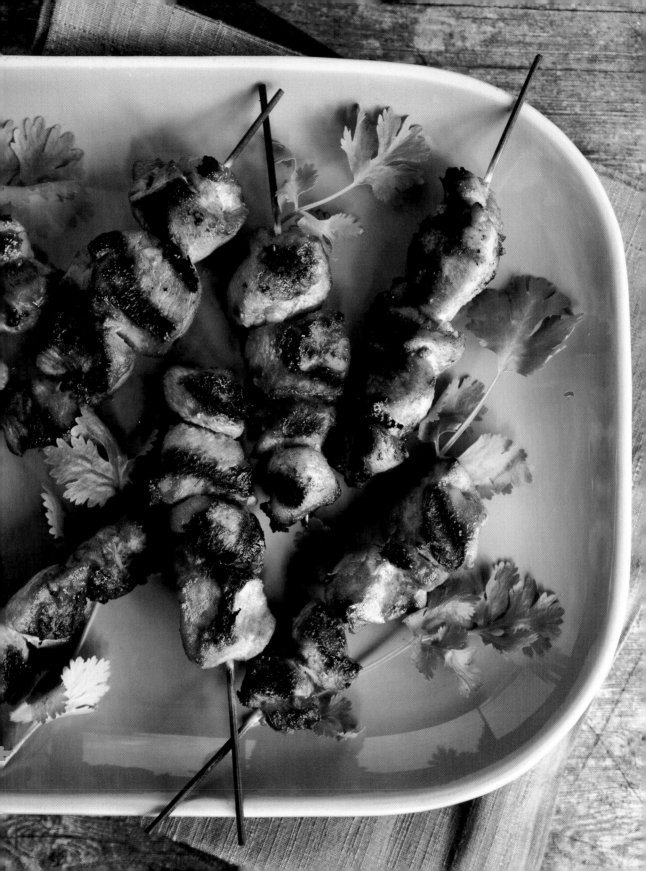

# Peanut Coconut Sauce

Some people love ketchup; others, barbecue sauce. In our home, this peanut coconut sauce is king. My daughter Abigail loves it so much that I often jokingly offer her some chicken with her sauce! She usually responds with a snarky grin, "More sauce, please."

**MAKES ALMOST 2 CUPS**

**One 13.5-ounce can coconut milk**

**¼ cup creamy peanut butter**

**¼ cup firmly packed dark brown sugar**

**1 tablespoon soy sauce**

**1½ teaspoons red curry paste**

Combine the coconut milk, peanut butter, brown sugar, soy sauce, and red curry paste in a saucepan and cook over medium heat for 3 minutes, stirring occasionally.

*Cook's note:* Use this sauce over grilled meat, vegetables, steamed rice, or your favorite pasta dish. It will keep for up to 2 weeks in the refrigerator.

*Note:* Chaokoh brand coconut milk works the best with this recipe because of its higher fat content, making for a thick and creamy sauce.

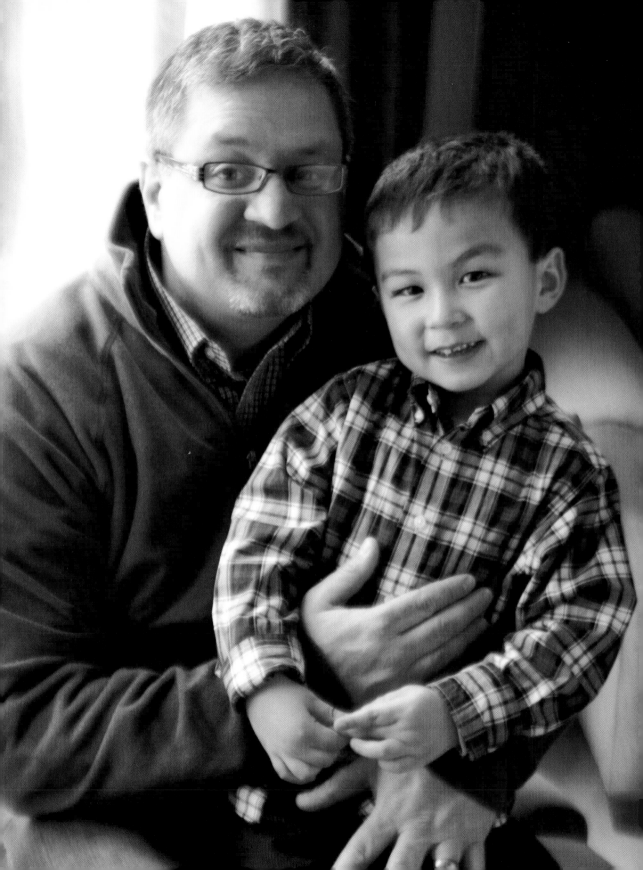

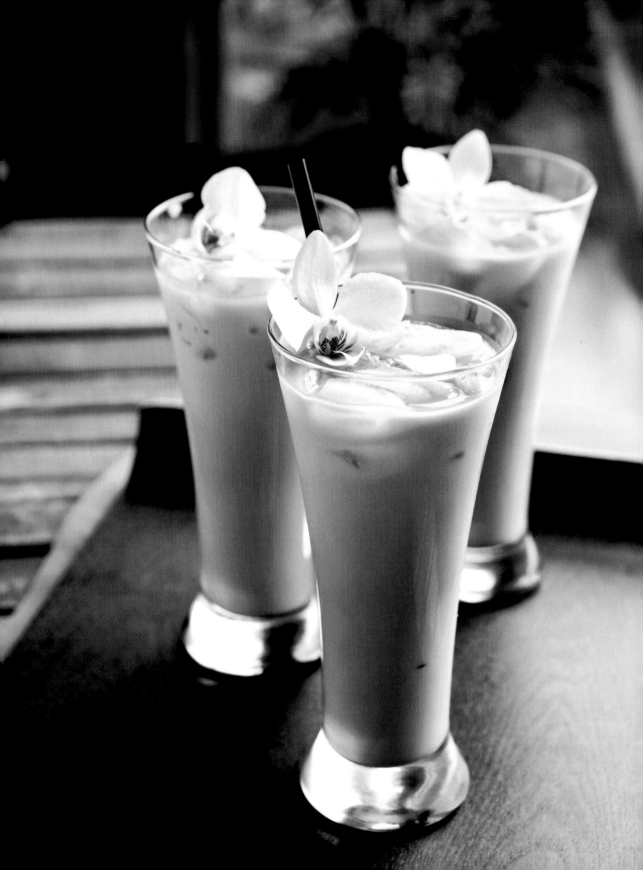

# Thai Iced Tea

When serving Asian food to family and friends, I love to include Thai iced tea to give our meal a more authentic flair—just like at a Thai restaurant. I often order this beverage when we eat out, but it's fun to make it at home too.

Combine the sugar, star anise, cinnamon sticks, and 6 cups of water in a medium saucepan, and bring to a boil. Add the tea bags and turn off the heat. Steep the tea for 5 minutes; then remove the star anise, cinnamon sticks, and tea bags. Let the tea cool completely; then stir in the sweetened condensed milk. Pour the tea into 6 ice-filled glasses, and serve each one with a straw.

*Just for fun:* For a richer flavor, substitute either orange spice or chai tea bags for half of the black tea bags.

**SERVES 6**

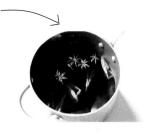

½ cup granulated sugar

6 whole star anise pods

3 small cinnamon sticks

10 black tea bags

½ cup sweetened condensed milk

Ice cubes

# six

# MIMI'S AFTERNOON TEA PARTY

My daughter Mimi has always loved hosting the most fabulous bedroom tea parties for her friends—both the human and the stuffed animal variety. I'm guessing this comes from the stories I've told her of my sisters and me having tea parties when we were kids. The food she serves during these impromptu afternoon teas consists of whatever she can find in the kitchen—PB&J sandwiches, nuts, cut fruit, cookies, and peach herbal tea, her favorite.

It's so stinking cute to eavesdrop on Mimi and her friends as they try their hardest to be sophisticated and well mannered, taking turns pouring tea into tiny porcelain cups on matching saucers and eating tiny bites with pinkies pointed up.

A few years ago I decided Mimi was old enough to start collecting real teacups. One year I bought her a full-size floral teapot made of porcelain china, and every year since I've given her a new cup and saucer for Christmas. I get so much joy out of watching her excitement with each new set she receives. I imagine someday she'll pass her collection down to her own daughter, but for now, they'll be displayed on a small white shelf in her bedroom for her to enjoy.

Every now and then I prepare a few special items and sit down beside her for tea. It's a treasured time for mom and daughter to share over a cup of tea and some cookies. I have a feeling Mimi and I will be sharing tea and stories long into her adulthood.

The recipes in this section are inspired by my precious afternoon tea dates with my daughter. The treats are intended to be savored slowly, with much chatting and sipping between bites. They can be prepared earlier in the day and then set aside for afternoon tea. All of them go nicely with traditional black tea or fruity herbal tea.

# Pint-Size Biscotti

Biscotti are one of my favorite coffee shop treats. I love that they aren't as sweet as cookies, yet still make the perfect dunking companion to my afternoon latte or tea. I'm convinced that people don't realize how easy these are to make. But that's okay with me; it will be our little secret.

**MAKES 18 BISCOTTI**

1 cup granulated sugar

2 eggs

¼ cup vegetable oil

1 tablespoon almond extract

¼ teaspoon ground or freshly grated nutmeg

2 cups all-purpose flour, plus more if needed

1 teaspoon baking powder

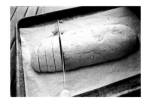

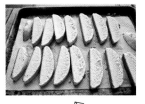

1. Preheat the oven to 375°F. Line a baking sheet with parchment paper.

2. In a medium bowl, combine the sugar, eggs, oil, almond extract, and nutmeg until well mixed. Add the flour and baking powder, and knead the mixture with your hands until a heavy, workable dough forms, adding more flour if necessary.

3. On a lightly floured surface, use your hands to shape and roll the dough into a 12-inch-long log. Transfer the log to the center of the baking sheet. Flatten the dough to form a ½-inch-thick rectangle that's a bit thicker in the center and thinner on the long sides.

4. Bake for 25 minutes, or until firm to the touch. Leaving the oven on, remove the biscotti loaf, on the parchment, place it on a cutting board, and let it cool for 5 to 8 minutes, until cool enough to touch but still warm.

5. Cut the loaf crosswise into ½-inch-thick slices. Place the slices on the baking sheet, lined with the parchment paper, cut side up, and bake for 8 minutes. Flip the biscotti over and bake for 8 minutes more. Let the biscotti cool completely on a wire rack before serving.

*Just for fun:* Melt 1 cup of chocolate chips and spread the chocolate sauce on a plate. Dip the flat bottom of each biscotti in the melted chocolate until the bottom is completely coated. Lay the biscotti on their sides on a cookie sheet and let the chocolate cool completely.

*Storing:* Store biscotti at room temperature in an airtight bag or plastic container for a week, or put in the freezer. Pull a piece out when you want one. Just be sure to let it sit at room temperature for about 10 minutes before eating.

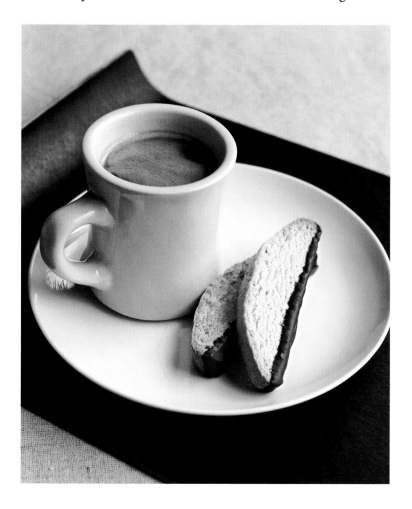

# Easy Strawberry Jam

If you've never made fresh strawberry jam, you're missing out on one of life's simplest pleasures. My kids love preparing jam from strawberries (or other berries) they've picked in our yard and then spreading some over small pats of butter on crusty French bread. And I love seeing their red-stained mouths and fingers as they lick off any traces of the jam because they know it's too good to waste.

**MAKES 1 CUP**

**2 cups chopped hulled fresh strawberries**

**1 cup granulated sugar**

**2 tablespoons fresh lemon juice**

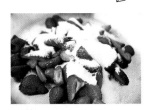
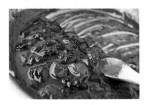

In a medium saucepan, cook the strawberries, sugar, and lemon juice over medium heat for about 20 minutes, stirring occasionally. The jam is ready when its consistency is like a thick maple syrup or the temperature reaches 220°F.

*Just for fun:* Substitute balsamic vinegar for the lemon juice for a rich, deep flavor. You can also swap in other berries along with the strawberries for a mixed berry variation.

*Storing:* This jam will keep in a sealed container in the refrigerator for up to 3 weeks. (A longer shelf life requires proper canning procedures and equipment.)

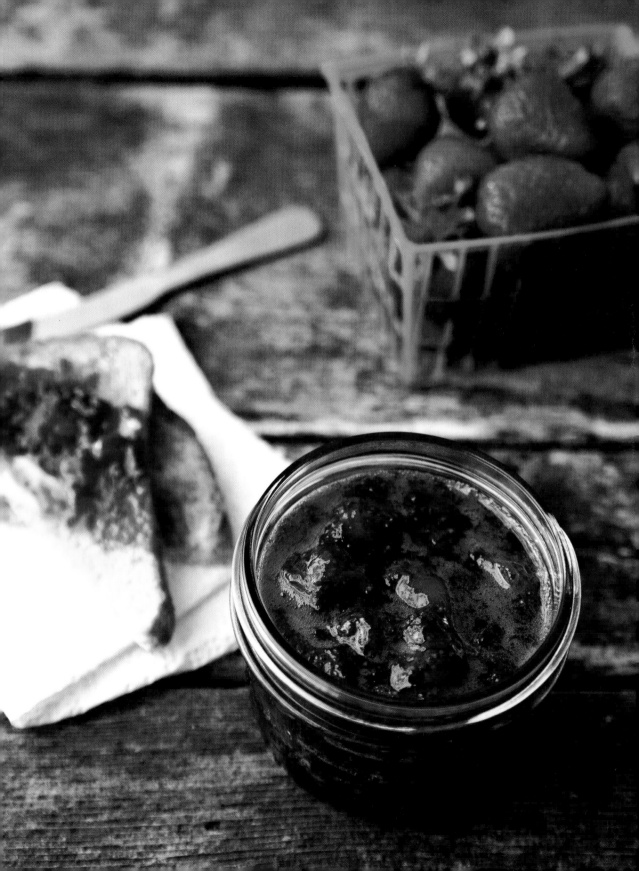

# Mini Thumbprint Jam Scones

These scones are so tender, they melt in your mouth—seriously. Lots of butter and heavy cream put these sweet tea biscuits in a class of their own. Just as with a thumbprint cookie, you get to taste a little bit of jam in every bite. Friends and family will rave about the drizzled almond glaze—a special finishing touch.

**MAKES 16 SCONES**

2½ cups all-purpose flour

⅓ cup granulated sugar

6 tablespoons (¾ stick) cold unsalted butter, cubed

1 tablespoon baking powder

½ teaspoon salt

1 cup heavy cream

1 egg, slightly beaten

2 teaspoons pure vanilla extract

½ cup jam (your favorite flavor)

¼ cup milk

1 cup confectioners' sugar

1 teaspoon almond extract

1. Preheat the oven to 400°F. Line a baking sheet with parchment paper.

2. Combine the flour, granulated sugar, butter, baking powder, and salt in a food processor, and pulse until a coarse meal forms. Transfer the mixture to a large mixing bowl. Add the heavy cream, egg, and vanilla, and knead the dough inside the bowl until it comes together. Divide the dough into 4 balls of equal size.

3. On a floured surface, flatten each ball of dough into a ¾-inch-thick disk. Cut each disk into 4 equal wedges. Place the wedges on the baking sheet, setting them 2 inches apart. Gently make a small indentation on top of each one with your thumb. Spoon a generous teaspoon of the jam into each indentation. Repeat with the remaining dough. Bake for 15 minutes, or until the bottoms are golden brown. Transfer the scones to a wire rack to cool.

4. While the scones are cooling, make the almond glaze: In a small microwave-safe bowl, heat the milk for 30 seconds. Slowly whisk in the confectioners' sugar and almond extract, whisking until the glaze is free of lumps.

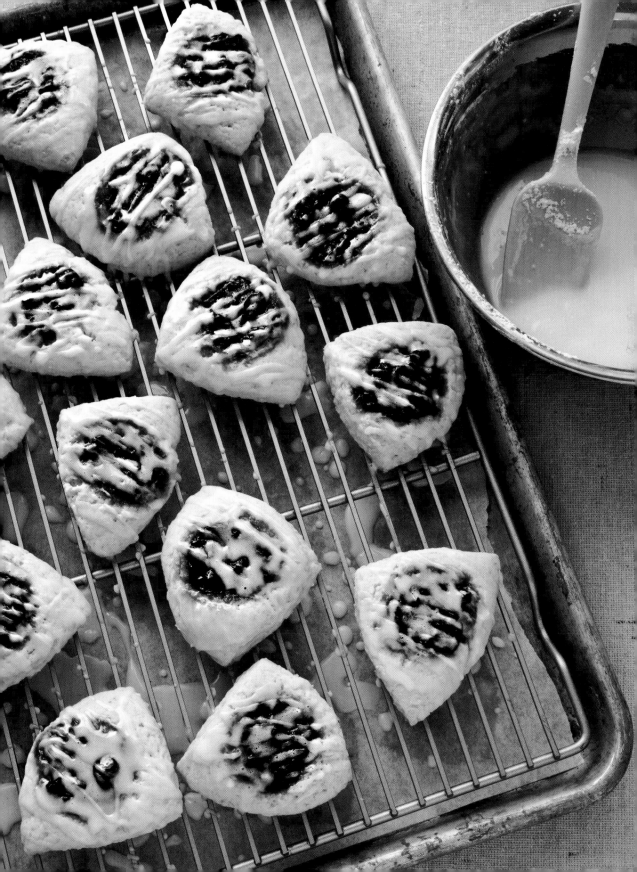

5. Dip a spoon into the glaze and drizzle the glaze over the scones. Let the glaze set for about 5 minutes before serving.

*No food processor?* Feel free to use your fingers to combine the ingredients until the mixture resembles coarse meal.

*Storing:* The scones will keep in a sealed container at room temperature for up to 3 days or in the freezer for up to 2 weeks.

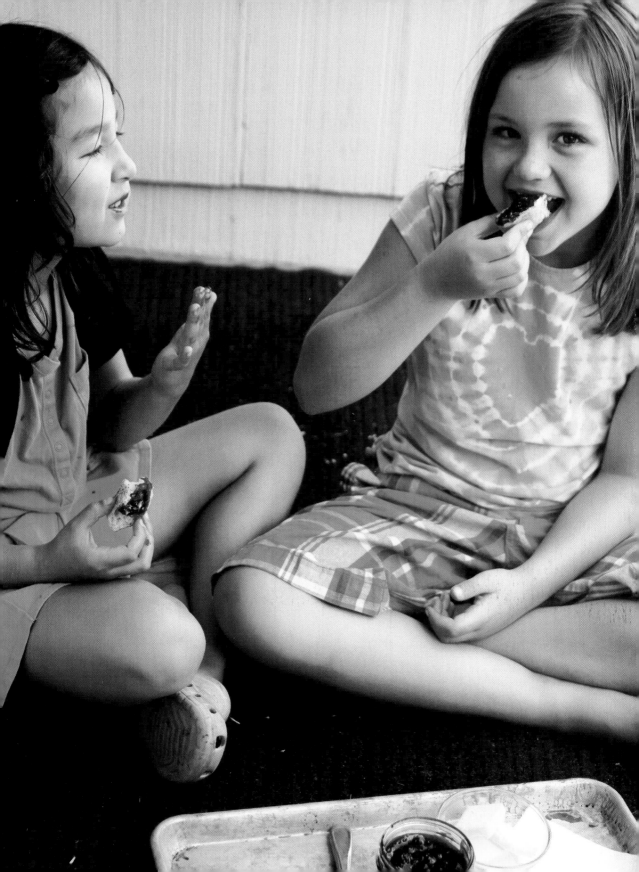

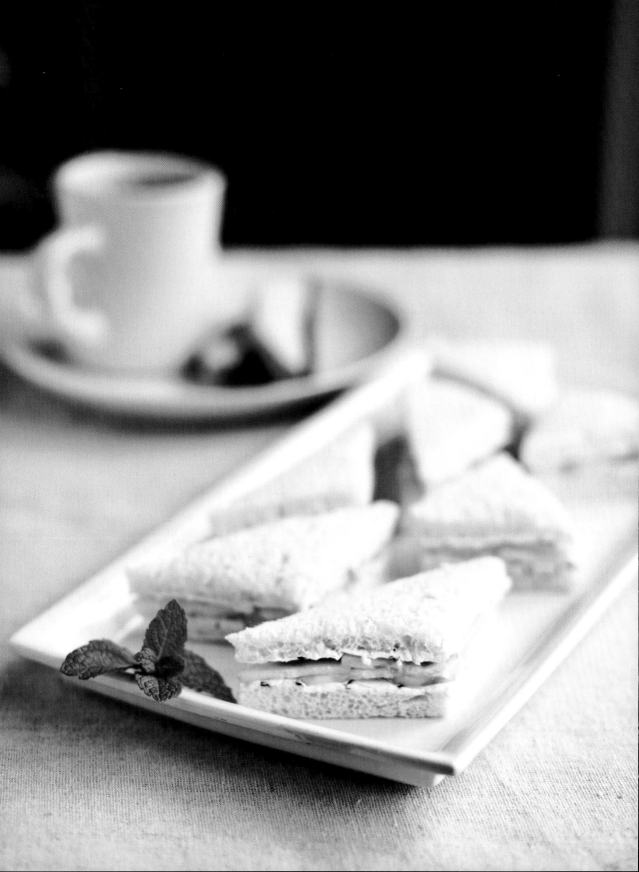

# Cucumber-Mint Tea Sandwiches

I'll never forget the first time my friend Leslie took me to Seattle's Queen Mary Tearoom, near University Village. While we drank tea and enjoyed our time together, we were treated to a delightful array of cookies, fruits, biscuits, and cucumber tea sandwiches served on dainty tiered trays. Since then, these refreshing cucumber-mint sandwiches have become a must-make at any tea party I host.

In a small bowl, combine the butter, cream cheese, and mint until thoroughly blended. Spread each slice of bread with the butter mixture. Evenly distribute the cucumber slices over the buttered sides of 4 slices of bread. Lightly season with salt, and top the sandwiches with the remaining slices of bread, buttered side down. Carefully cut and discard the crusts from each sandwich. Cut each sandwich diagonally into quarters.

*Variation:* Substitute dill for the mint for a completely different but pleasant flavor. Since dill is commonly used for pickling vegetables, it adds a subtle pickle-like flavor to the cream cheese.

**MAKES 16 TEA SANDWICHES**

**5 tablespoons unsalted butter, at room temperature**

**5 tablespoons cream cheese, at room temperature**

**¼ cup finely chopped fresh mint**

**8 slices white bread**

**One 6-inch piece seedless cucumber, peeled and thinly sliced**

**Salt**

# Pretty in Pink Marshmallow Pops

Like millions of people, I'm a big fan of Bakerella's (Angie Dudley's) creative cake pops—a mixture of crumbled cake and frosting on a stick, coated in chocolate or other flavors and cleverly decorated with sprinkles and candy. Inspired by her bite-size desserts, these marshmallow pops are easy to make and have a cuteness factor of 10. If you're looking for an easy treat to prepare for birthday parties, baby and bridal showers, or party favors, these marshmallow pops are a perfect choice.

**MAKES 36 POPS**

*Special equipment:*
**36 lollipop sticks, Styrofoam block**

**16 ounces pink candy coating**

**1 package large marshmallows**

**White nonpareils (sprinkles)**

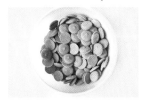

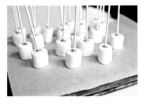

1. Following the directions on the package, melt the candy coating in a medium bowl until it is smooth. Dip the tip of a lollipop stick ¼ inch deep in the candy coating. Insert the dipped end of the stick into the center of the flat side of a marshmallow, about three-quarters of the way in. Place the marshmallow on a cookie sheet with the stick pointed upward. Repeat with the rest of the marshmallows.

2. Dip a marshmallow pop into the candy coating, turning it gently until it is fully coated. Lift the marshmallow pop straight up from the candy coating and tilt the pop so that the excess coating drips back into the bowl. With the pop in one hand, use the index finger of the other hand to gently tap the lollipop stick until there's no excess candy coating. Carefully hold the marshmallow pop over a plate and sprinkle the nonpareils onto the pop while rotating the stick. Stick the ends of the lollipop sticks into the Styrofoam block to dry. Repeat with the rest of the lollipops.

3. The pops can be individually wrapped in food-grade plastic gusset bags of the kind used to package lollipops and candy.

*Cook's note:* Candy coating wafers also come in different colors including blue, orange, red, green, white, and chocolate flavored. Unused wafers can be stored in a sealed bag. Any remaining leftover melted wafers should be discarded.

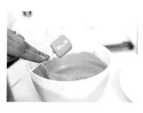

*Just for fun:* Feel free to use sprinkles or decorative sugar instead of the nonpareils. Just make sure you don't use any heavy toppings, which could pull off the candy coating.

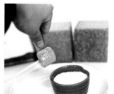

*Where to buy:* Candy coating, lollipop sticks, Styrofoam blocks, and gusset bags can be purchased at cake and candy supply stores, or at craft stores such as Michaels.

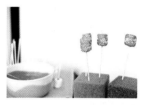

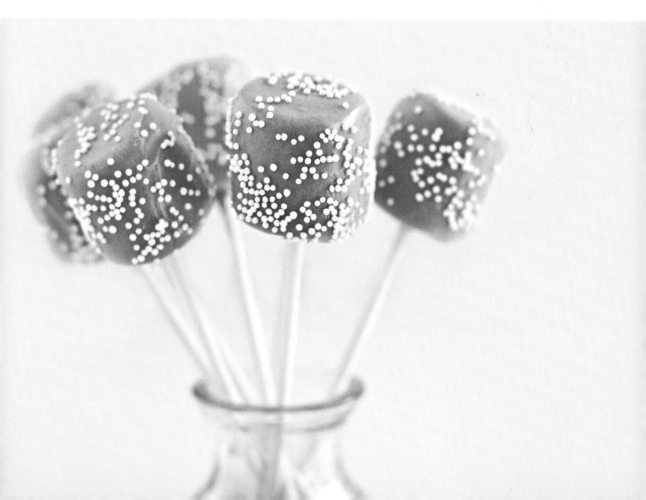

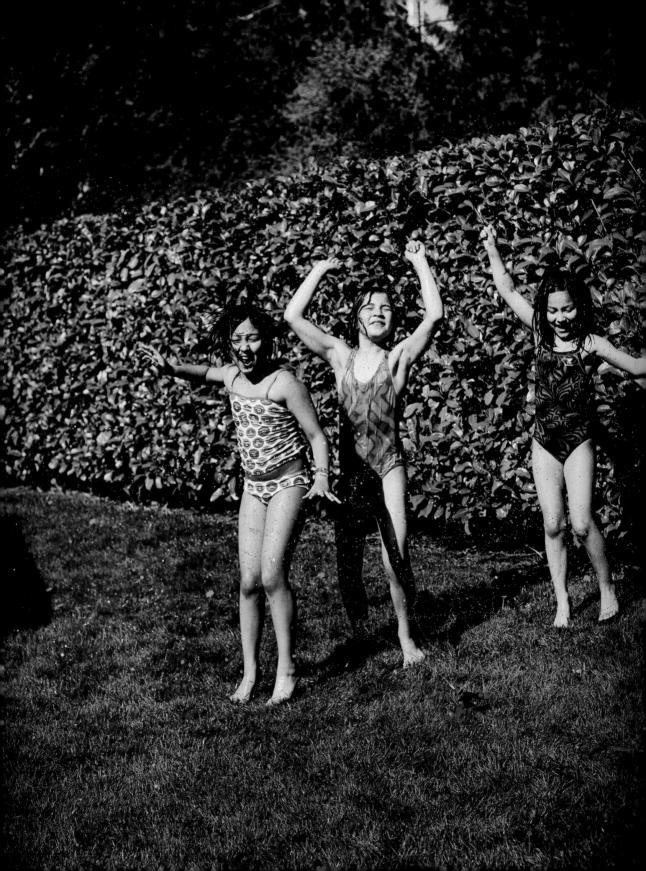

# seven

# BLOCK PARTY

I love the scene in the movie *The Sandlot* where the neighbors gather outside on July 4th with their decorated tables filled with foods of every kind. Kids are riding bikes, goofing off, and enjoying the moment as they wait for darkness to fall and fireworks to light up the evening sky.

Every year our neighborhood has a block party and each family brings a dish to share. Card tables are neatly arranged side by side on someone's lawn, and chairs line the driveway like an airport runway. Beach towels and picnic blankets are spread out over several lawns while neighbors chat about the latest news and what their kids have been up to.

Don't even get me started on the food! I'm always eager to eat someone else's home cooking, and I love sharing my favorite dishes with others. It's amazing how the power of food can bring neighbors closer together and help build a strong sense of community. From macaroni salad to blackberry crisp, these memorable dishes will be appreciated—and anticipated—at future get-togethers.

# Hawaiian Plate Lunch Macaroni Salad

When we go on vacation on the island of Oahu, I love to eat as the locals do, cooling off with a rainbow shaved ice from Waiola's or eating a slice of Ted's Bakery's chocolate haupia pie. And Hawaiian plate lunches are our take-alongs for a day at the beach. A typical plate lunch consists of rice, meat, and a scoop of macaroni salad. This recipe is inspired by all the different plate lunches I've had the pleasure of eating. Aloha!

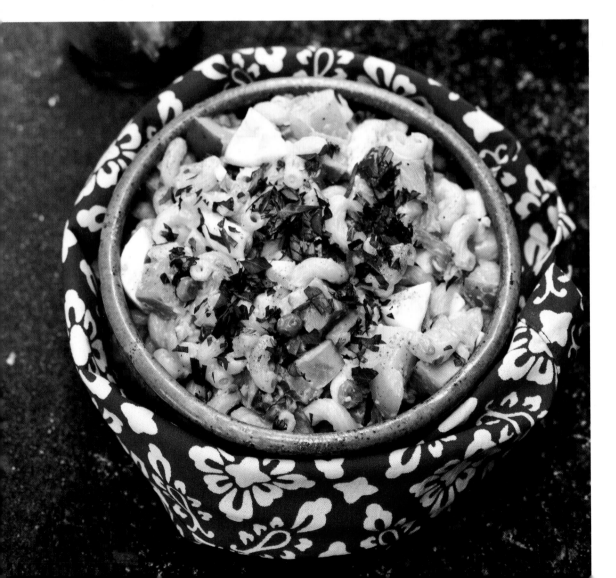

1. Bring 2 large saucepans of salted water to a boil.

2. Cut the potatoes into 1-inch cubes. Add them to one pot of boiling water and simmer until fork-tender, about 8 minutes. Drain well and set aside.

3. Cook the elbow macaroni in the second saucepan of boiling water until al dente, according to the directions on the package. Drain well, and set aside.

4. Transfer the potatoes and pasta to a large salad bowl. Add all the remaining ingredients and toss well. Add more seasoned salt and black pepper if necessary. Cover, and refrigerate the salad until ready to serve.

*Cook's note:* This macaroni salad is perfect for large gatherings and potlucks. Feel free to halve the recipe to serve it as part of a regular family dinner. Leftovers make a great side dish in a packed lunch, too!

*Time-saving tip:* Forget the chopping! Many of the ingredients in this recipe can be found at your grocery store's salad bar.

SERVES 12 AS
A SIDE DISH

1 pound red or Yukon Gold potatoes, scrubbed and peeled

One 16-ounce package elbow macaroni

1½ cups mayonnaise (I like Best Foods or Hellmann's)

3 celery ribs, chopped

2 carrots, peeled and grated

3 hard-boiled eggs, chopped

½ pound ham, cut into ⅓-inch cubes

½ cup frozen peas

½ cup chopped dill pickles

¼ cup finely chopped red onion

2 teaspoons seasoned salt (I like Lawry's), or more if needed

½ teaspoon freshly ground black pepper, or more if needed

# Fiesta Corn Salad

If you're looking for an easy recipe for your next outdoor gathering, it doesn't get much simpler than this. With a little bit of whisking, chopping, and tossing, this colorful salad is the perfect side dish for easy entertaining.

**SERVES 6 TO 8**

¼ cup fresh lime juice

2 tablespoons extra-virgin olive oil

2 garlic cloves, minced

1½ teaspoons ground cumin

¼ teaspoon cayenne pepper

4 cups frozen corn kernels

One 14-ounce can black beans, rinsed and drained

1 red bell pepper, seeded and chopped

¼ cup chopped fresh cilantro

Salt and freshly ground black pepper

1. In a large bowl, whisk together the lime juice, olive oil, garlic, cumin, and cayenne. Add the corn, black beans, and red bell pepper, and mix gently until just incorporated. Cover and chill for 1 hour.

2. Just before serving, add the cilantro, season with salt and pepper, and toss.

*Cook's note:* This salad can be served as a side dish, or with tortilla chips as a salsa-like condiment.

*Just for fun:* Add 2 cups of cooked bow-tie pasta and ½ cup of halved cherry tomatoes for a delicious pasta salad.

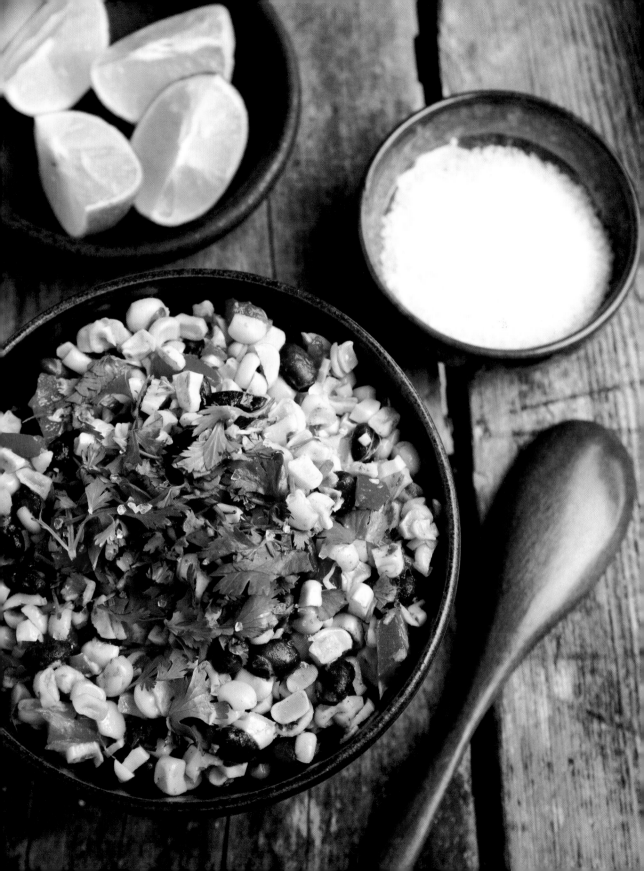

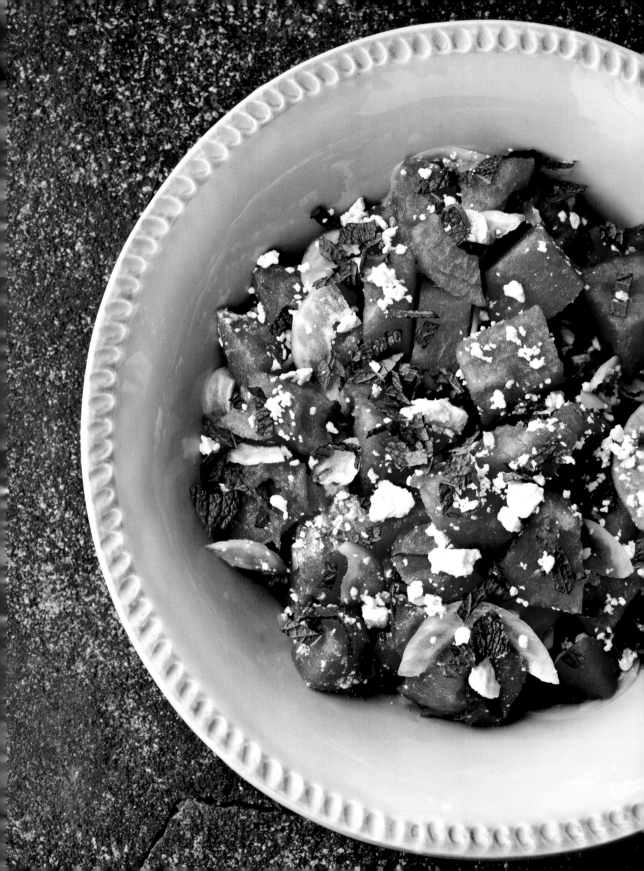

# Watermelon Feta Salad

For one moment allow me to declare myself a watermelon feta salad evangelist. *You need to make this salad!* I know it sounds odd to pair refreshing, juicy watermelon with onions and feta cheese, but I promise you, it's surprisingly good. In fact, it's so good you may find yourself eating seconds and probably thirds.

Combine the watermelon, feta cheese, red onion, and mint in a large bowl. Pour the lime juice and the olive oil over the watermelon mixture, and toss gently to coat. Serve immediately.

*Cook's note:* Don't be tempted to prepare this salad in advance, other than prepping the individual ingredients. If the salad is made before you're ready to serve it, the feta cheese will start to turn mushy and will make this beautiful salad look unappetizing.

**SERVES 6 TO 8**

**6 cups cubed watermelon**

**1 cup crumbled feta cheese**

**¼ cup thinly sliced red onion**

**¼ cup chopped fresh mint**

**¼ cup fresh lime juice**

**1 tablespoon extra-virgin olive oil**

# Blackberry Crisp

I have a love-hate relationship with the invasive blackberry brambles taking over my backyard. Every year I cut them back, and the following season they grow back more fiercely and even more widespread. The only consolation I have is the bountiful blackish purple berries they produce. When life gives you blackberries, make blackberry crisp!

**SERVES 12 TO 16**

¾ cup granulated sugar

2 teaspoons cornstarch

6 cups blackberries (fresh or frozen)

Juice of 1 lemon

¾ cup all-purpose flour

¾ cup firmly packed dark brown sugar

8 tablespoons (1 stick) cold unsalted butter, cut into ½-inch cubes

1 cup rolled oats

Vanilla ice cream, for serving

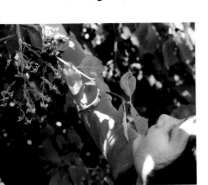

1. Preheat the oven to 400°F. Spray a 9 x 13-inch baking dish with nonstick cooking spray.

2. In a large bowl, mix the sugar and cornstarch. Add the blackberries and lemon juice, and toss gently with the sugar. Transfer the blackberries to the baking dish.

3. Combine the flour, brown sugar, and butter in a food processor, and pulse until the mixture resembles coarse meal. (If you don't have a food processor, work the mixture with your hands by rubbing the ingredients between your thumb and fingers.) Place the mixture in a large zip-top plastic bag. Add the oats and mix all the ingredients by sealing the bag and shaking it for a few seconds. Sprinkle the mixture over the berries.

4. Bake for 45 minutes, or until the topping is slightly browned. Serve the crisp hot or cold, with a scoop of vanilla ice cream.

*Just for fun:* For a great seasonal summer dessert, consider substituting sliced fresh peaches for half of the blackberries.

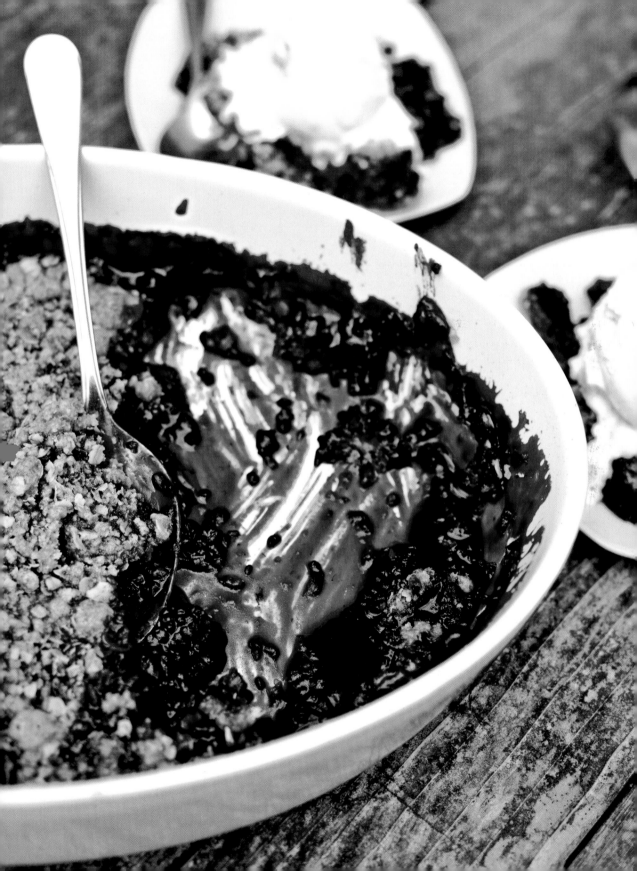

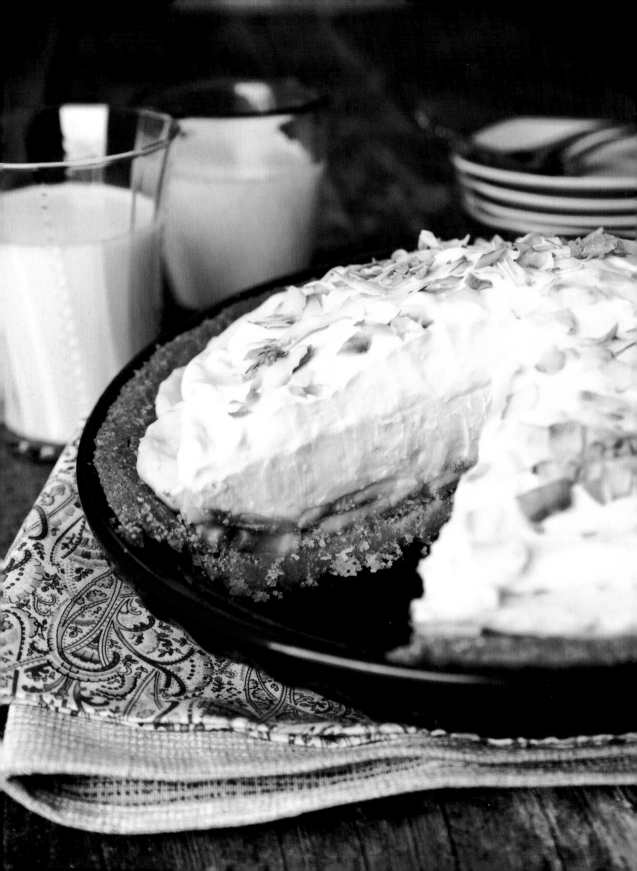

# Banana Cream Pie

Who doesn't love banana cream pie? Here's my simplified version of this classic, which is one of my most requested desserts to bring to family gatherings. It features a thick coconut cookie crust, which is a nice twist on the traditional pie crust. Each time I bring this to a party, at least one person asks me for the recipe.

1. Preheat the oven to 350°F. Spray a 9-inch pie plate with nonstick cooking spray.

2. To make the crust, combine the cookie crumbs, sugar, salt, and butter in a medium bowl, and mix by hand until the crumbs look moist. Press the crumb mixture evenly over the bottom and sides of the pie plate. Bake for 12 to 15 minutes, until golden brown. Set aside to cool completely. Don't worry if the cookie crust seems soft; it will harden as it cools.

3. To make the filling, arrange the banana slices in layers on the bottom of the cooled crust, and set aside. In a large cold bowl, mix the powdered pudding mixes, 1 cup of the heavy cream, and the milk on medium speed until the mixture has the consistency of a thick custard. Spread the pudding evenly over the bananas.

4. In a medium cold bowl, combine the remaining 1 cup heavy cream, the vanilla extract, and the confectioners' sugar. Whip on medium-high speed until firm peaks form. Spread the sweetened whipped cream over the pudding layer. Sprinkle the toasted coconut flakes over the top, and refrigerate for at least 1 hour before serving.

*Cook's note:* Refrigerating the pie helps it to set up, so it will slice beautifully when it's time to serve it.

**SERVES 8**

**CRUST**

1½ cups coconut cookie crumbs (I use Mother's Coconut Cocadas)

⅓ cup granulated sugar

½ teaspoon salt

6 tablespoons (¾ stick) unsalted butter, melted

**FILLING**

2 ripe bananas, cut into ¼-inch-thick disks

½ box (3.4-ounce box) Jell-O vanilla instant pudding

½ box (3.4-ounce box) Jell-O banana instant pudding

2 cups heavy cream

1 cup whole milk

2 teaspoons pure vanilla extract

¾ cup confectioners' sugar

½ cup shredded sweetened or unsweetened coconut, toasted

I've made this pie using different brands of instant pudding, and I've found that Jell-O brand tastes best because of its subtle flavoring.

*Just for fun:* Feel free to add 2 tablespoons of bourbon to the whipped cream topping for a special added touch. Sometimes I also like to drizzle ¼ cup of caramel sauce on top!

*Make ahead:* This pie can be made 24 hours in advance; any longer and you'll have a soggy crust. Just be sure to loosely cover the pie with plastic wrap before refrigerating it.

*eight*

# SUMMER FUN
# IN THE SUN

Happiness is exuberant kids running through a sprinkler and being chased with a garden hose, squealing and laughing in the warmth of a hot summer day. A day of summer fun would not be complete without short breaks to enjoy a creamy mango frozen yogurt pop or a nice tall glass of refreshing strawberry lemonade. This is what summer is all about.

When evening sets in, we like to invite a few of the neighborhood kids over for an outdoor movie. Rob hooks up his laptop and projector in the backyard and completes his makeshift outdoor theater by nailing a white king-size bed sheet to our woodshed. The kids lay their sleeping bags and pillows on the grass and claim their favorite viewing spot. While Rob handles the technical details of the evening, I focus my energy on the snacks. To make these evenings extra fun and special, I can be found in the kitchen pouring fizzy root beer floats, seasoning big bowls of zesty popcorn, and making a batch of gooey oven-broiled s'mores.

While the movie is playing, Rob and I sit in the back with our own bowl of popcorn and adult treats—daiquiri lime ice pops—as we relish having "that house," the one where kids come to have fun and leave feeling special.

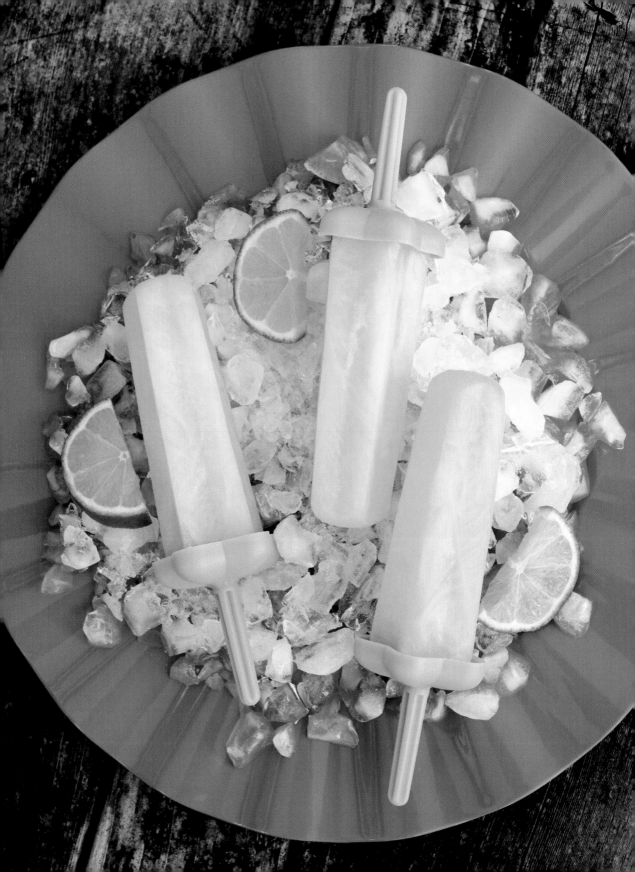

# Daiquiri Lime Ice Pops

Nothing beats the cool and refreshing taste of citrus drinks or ice-cold treats on a hot summer day. When the weather justifies the need for tank tops, shorts, and flip-flops, I start making my favorite ice pops. Inspired by Baskin Robbins' Daiquiri Ice sorbet, these pops are a fun alternative for adult summertime guests.

1. In a medium saucepan over medium-low heat, bring the sugar, lime juice, and 1½ cups water to a simmering boil. Stir until the sugar dissolves. Remove the pan from the heat and stir in the rum and food coloring. Cool the mixture, then pour it into ice-pop molds. Cover the opening of each mold with a small piece of foil, and insert a pop stick halfway into the mold. Freeze overnight.

2. To release a pop from the mold, carefully hold the pop in one hand while running warm water over the mold without getting water into the opening. With the other hand, gently pull the stick away from the mold until the ice pop releases.

**MAKES 4 TO 6 POPS**

*Special equipment:* **ice-pop molds, wooden pop sticks**

**1 cup granulated sugar**

**½ cup fresh lime juice**

**2 tablespoons rum**

**1 or 2 drops green food coloring**

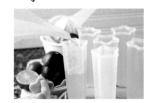

# Mango Frozen Yogurt Pops

Inspired by mango lassi, a popular East Indian drink, these are one of my favorite treats to serve my kids. I get a sense of motherly satisfaction when I offer these all-natural, healthy, frozen yogurt pops to the kids and their friends. I love the combination of creamy yogurt and fruit and could eat several of these, one right after the other, without an ounce of guilt.

**MAKES 4 TO 6 POPS**

*Special equipment:*
**ice-pop molds, wooden pop sticks**

**12 ounces fresh ripe or frozen mangoes, cut into chunks**

**1 cup orange juice**

**One 6-ounce container vanilla Greek yogurt**

**¾ cup granulated sugar**

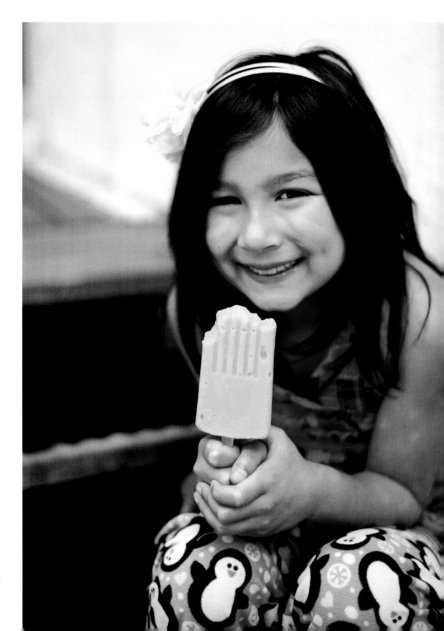

1. Combine all the ingredients in a blender, and blend until smooth. Pour the yogurt mixture into the ice-pop molds. Cover the opening of each mold with a small piece of foil, and insert a wooden pop stick halfway into each one. Freeze overnight.

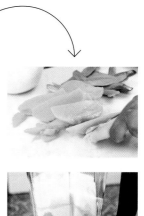

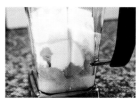

2. To release a pop from the mold, carefully hold the pop in one hand while running warm water over the mold without getting water into the opening. With the other hand, gently pull the wooden stick away from the mold until the ice pop releases.

*Variations:* Frozen blueberries, strawberries, bananas, peaches, and raspberries can be substituted for the mango.

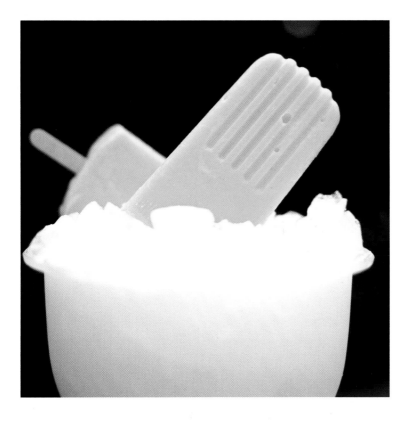

# Strawberry Lemonade

Our friends love it when I serve this easy strawberry lemonade. Using two store-bought ingredients, this refreshing drink can be made in seconds and is guaranteed to vanish quickly at any gathering.

**MAKES 10 CUPS**

**One 64-ounce carton all-natural lemonade**

**One 16-ounce container frozen sliced strawberries with sugar, thawed**

**Ice cubes**

**Lemon slices (optional)**

Combine the lemonade and strawberries in a large pitcher. Serve in cups filled with ice. Garnish with lemon slices if desired.

*Not sweet enough?* Add a second container of the sweetened sliced strawberries if you prefer your lemonade super sweet.

*Adult variation:* Add 1 ounce of vodka to every glass for a "hard" version of this classic summer drink.

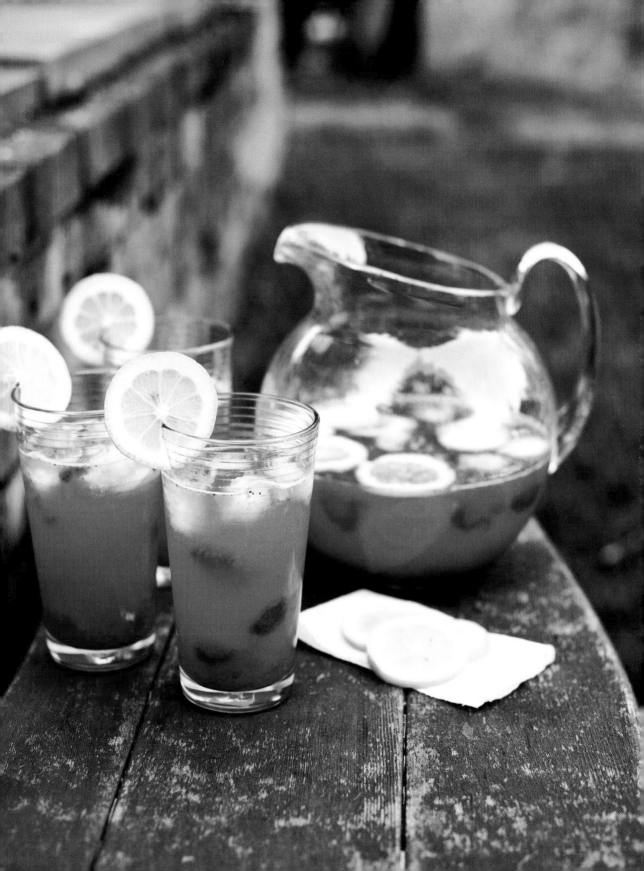

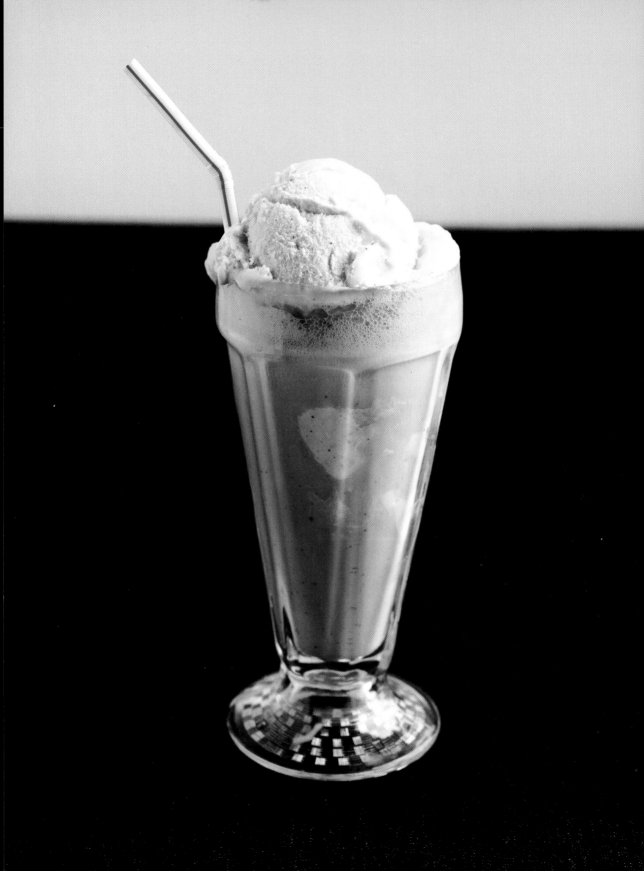

# Old-Fashioned Root Beer Floats

There's something magical and nostalgic about root beer floats that has carried through the generations. Watching the foamy fizz rise when root beer hits the vanilla ice cream invokes childlike excitement at any age. My kids and I love making root beer floats for a chilly, thirst-quenching summertime ice cream treat.

Fill 4 tall glasses with 2 scoops of vanilla ice cream each. Slowly pour half a bottle of root beer into each glass, making sure to stop when the foam reaches the top of the glass and wait for it to recede before pouring more. Serve with a straw and a spoon.

*Just for fun:* Top off each float with whipped cream and a maraschino cherry.

**MAKES 4 SERVINGS**

**1 pint vanilla ice cream**

**Two 12-ounce bottles old-fashioned root beer soda**

# Parmesan Ranch Popcorn

I love seasoned popcorn. The combination of Parmesan cheese and ranch flavoring is a guilty pleasure of mine. This is the perfect anytime snack, but a must-have for your next movie night!

**MAKES 16 CUPS**

**2 tablespoons grated Parmesan cheese**

**1 teaspoon dry ranch dressing mix**

**1 teaspoon salt**

**½ cup popcorn kernels**

**4 tablespoons (½ stick) unsalted butter, melted**

1. Combine the grated Parmesan, ranch dressing mix, and salt in a bowl.

2. Pop the popcorn kernels according to your air popper's manual, and pour them into a large bowl. Drizzle half the melted butter over the popcorn. Gently toss the popcorn with a circular motion to distribute the butter. Drizzle the remaining butter over the popcorn and toss again. Sprinkle the Parmesan seasoning over the popcorn, and toss gently one more time before serving.

*Just for fun:* If you like your popcorn on the spicier side, add up to ½ teaspoon of ground chipotle or cayenne pepper to the mix.

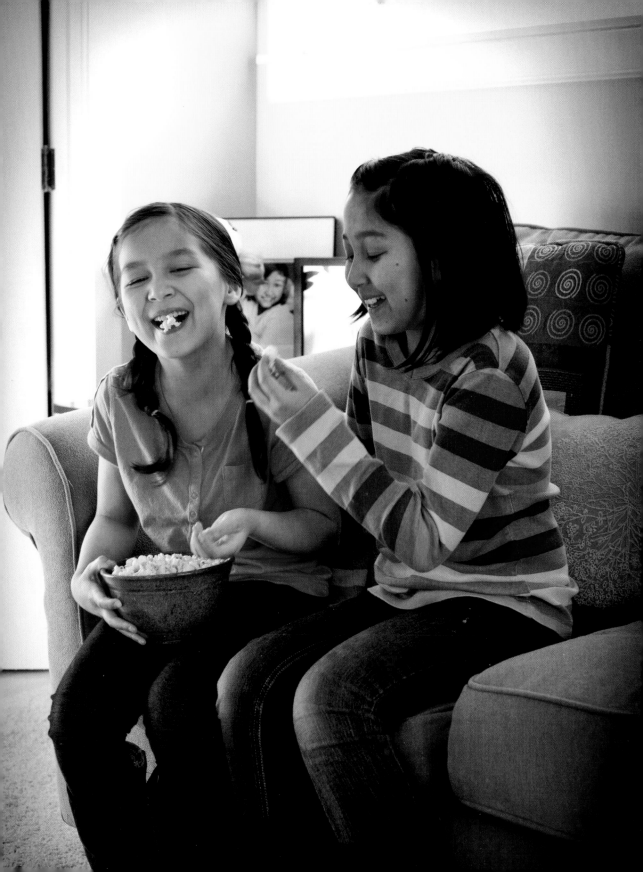

# Oven-Broiled S'mores

Making this classic campfire treat at home became so much easier once I realized I could broil a big batch of them in the oven, using the broiler. The marshmallows turn out gooey with a slightly golden crust and the chocolate is perfectly melted. This method makes it easy for you to enjoy s'mores from the comfort of your home. They also make great cookies and classroom treats!

**MAKES 24 S'MORES**

**One 14- to 16-ounce box graham crackers**

**One 10-ounce bag mini marshmallows**

**One 12-ounce bag semisweet chocolate chips**

1. Position an oven rack two notches down from the top, and set the oven to broil. Line a baking sheet with parchment paper.

2. Snap all the graham crackers into 2-cracker squares. Place half the cracker squares in rows on the baking sheet, without any gaps. Spread the mini marshmallows evenly across the graham crackers, followed by the chocolate chips.

3. Place the baking sheet in the oven, leaving the door slightly ajar. Broil the s'mores for approximately 5 minutes, or until the marshmallows have a nice golden brown edge. Make sure to keep an eye on them so that they don't burn.

4. Remove the baking sheet from the oven and quickly place the remaining graham cracker squares on top of the broiled s'mores. Press each square down gently but firmly enough that the marshmallow sticks to the top graham cracker. Allow them to cool for a few minutes before serving.

*Cook's note:* If you would like to serve these as regular cookies, allow the s'mores to cool for at least an hour. Then gently pull the square crackers apart from each other, just enough so that you can cut through the marshmallow strands with kitchen shears. The graham crackers will be nice and crunchy and the marshmallow filling will be firm but chewy. The chocolate will be hardened but tastes great.

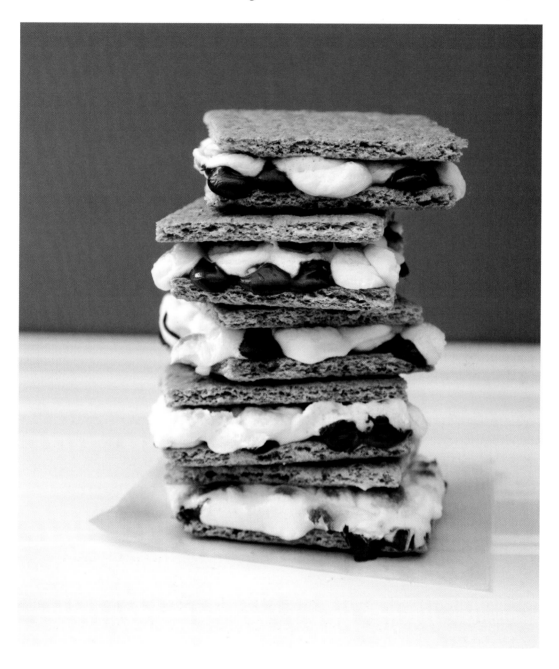

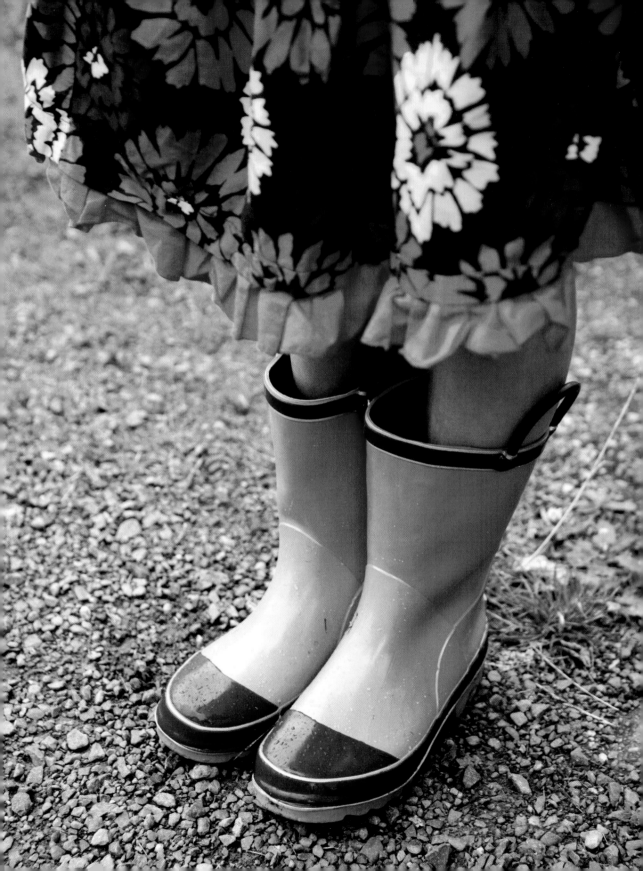

# nine

# POTLUCKS

Everyone loves a good potluck. The idea of eating tasty bites of other people's cooking is always exciting to me, except when I see a serving table with six variations of the same dish. Don't get me wrong—I love lasagna and spaghetti. I just prefer not to eat them six different ways in one sitting.

To avoid falling into the dreaded lasagna trap, I used to search cookbooks and the Internet for impressive (and often complicated) recipes I thought would wow others. Like many people, I would wait until the day of the party to prepare a dish for the first time, then cross my fingers and hope the guests would enjoy it. It was like throwing a Hail Mary pass at the end of a football game—risky and hardly ever successful. Not only were the dishes rarely appetizing, but at the end of the party I would leave with a barely touched dish showing only the outline of my husband's courtesy scoop, which I'm not even convinced he ate.

Now when I receive an invitation to a potluck, I always stick with my tried-and-true dishes. And I know that they're crowd-pleasers because I'm usually approached for the recipes during the course of the party. This is the ultimate potluck compliment, though having my dishes devoured first is a close second—no more doing the walk of shame with a full casserole dish.

The recipes in this chapter are surefire hits for any group gathering. They're always well received, first to disappear, and requested again and again.

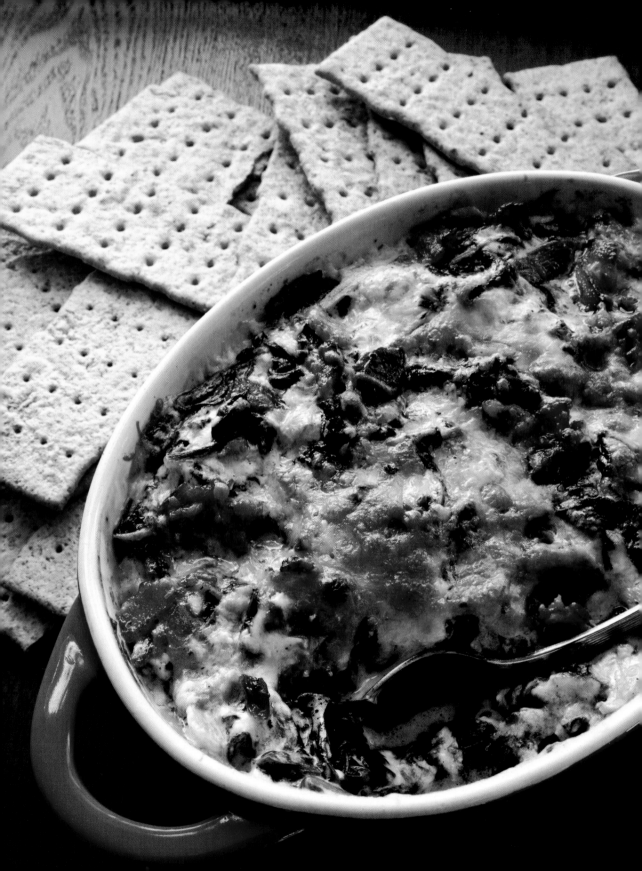

# Spicy Bacon Spinach Artichoke Dip

I love making this dip when company comes over or when I'm asked to bring a dish to a party. It's so delicious and addicting, I dare you to eat only one spoonful!

1. Preheat the oven to 400°F.

2. Heat the frozen spinach in the microwave for 5 minutes. Carefully squeeze out as much water as possible and set aside.

3. Microwave the cream cheese for 1 minute. Combine the cream cheese, mayonnaise, sour cream, cayenne, and garlic powder in a large bowl, and blend together well. Add the spinach, bacon, artichoke hearts, and both cheeses. Stir all the ingredients together until everything is well combined.

4. Spread the mixture out in a pie or tart plate or in a small casserole dish. Bake for 30 minutes, or until bubbling and slightly browned on top.

5. Serve hot with crackers, pita crisps, or vegetable sticks, or inside a hollowed-out sourdough bread with the cubed bread on the side.

*Serving idea:* Divide the mixture among smaller baking dishes or ramekins before baking it. Place the dishes of the cooked dip in different areas of the house for your party.

*Shopping tip:* Look in the cheese section at the grocery store for an 8-ounce bag of shredded cheese called "Italian." This blend is made of 1 cup of Parmesan and 1 cup of mozzarella cheese—exactly what this recipe calls for.

**MAKES 5 CUPS**

One 10-ounce package frozen chopped spinach

One 8-ounce package cream cheese

½ cup mayonnaise

½ cup sour cream

3 teaspoons cayenne pepper

2 teaspoons garlic powder

1 pound bacon, cooked and crumbled

One 14-ounce can artichoke hearts, drained and coarsely chopped

1 cup grated Parmesan cheese

1 cup shredded mozzarella cheese

# Chop Chop Salad

I love salads that have a variety of textures and flavors, along with the perfect dressing to bring out the best in each ingredient. This trendy Italian salad has it all and can be served as a main course or alongside your favorite pasta dish with a glass of wine. It also complements a slice of pizza very nicely!

**SERVES 4 TO 6**

**DRESSING**

¼ cup red wine vinegar

1 tablespoon Dijon mustard

½ teaspoon kosher salt

Freshly ground black pepper

½ cup olive oil

**SALAD**

1 head green leaf lettuce, chopped

½ pound salami, cut into ½-inch cubes

½ cup drained canned garbanzo beans (chickpeas)

½ cup shredded provolone cheese

½ cup chopped seeded red bell pepper

½ cup chopped red onion

In a small bowl, whisk all the dressing ingredients together. Just before serving, toss the salad ingredients with the dressing in a large salad bowl.

*Variation:* For a salad with a deeper, bolder, sweeter flavor, substitute balsamic vinegar for the red wine vinegar and omit the Dijon mustard.

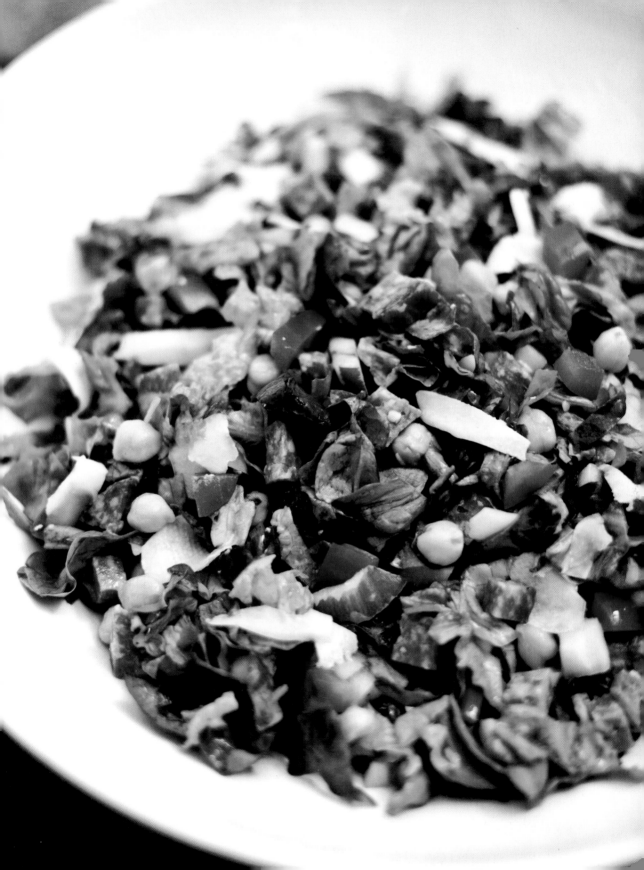

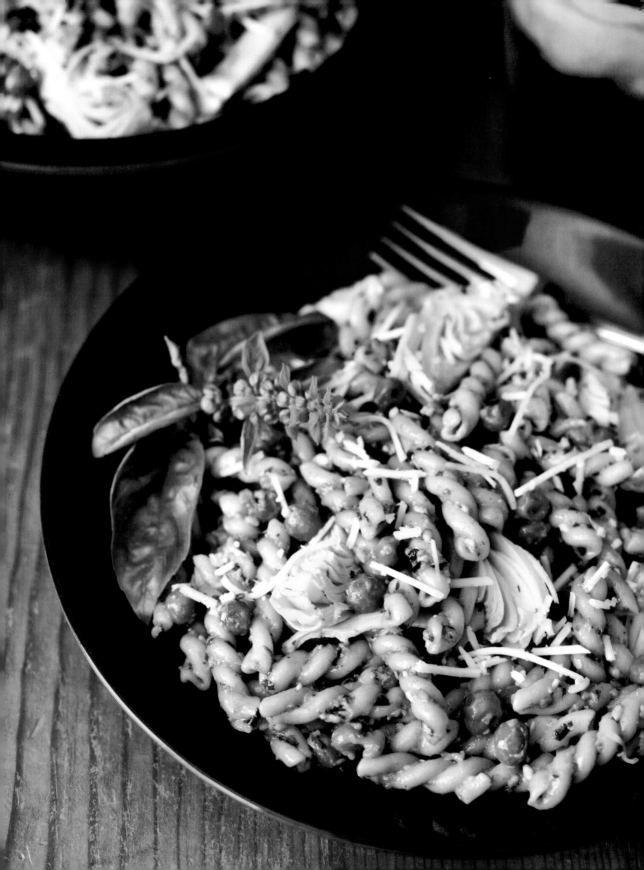

# Creamy Pesto Pasta Salad

This recipe is inspired by one of my favorite restaurants, Pagliacci Pizza. I've been eating their pesto pasta salad since I was in middle school and have now perfected my own version. Best served cold, this salad is equally tasty the next day.

**SERVES 6**

1 cup Basil Pesto
(recipe follows)

½ cup mayonnaise

One 16-ounce box fusilli pasta

1 cup frozen peas

One 14-ounce can artichoke hearts, drained and quartered

½ cup freshly grated Parmesan cheese

1. In a small bowl, combine the pesto and the mayonnaise; set aside.

2. Bring a large pot of salted water to a boil. Add the fusilli and cook until al dente, following the package directions.

3. Drain the pasta and transfer it to a large bowl. Add the frozen peas and the pesto dressing, and toss until well mixed and coated. Gently fold in the artichoke hearts. Chill the salad, covered, in the refrigerator for 20 minutes.

4. Sprinkle the Parmesan cheese over the salad just prior to serving.

*Make it a meal:* Add 2 cups cubed cooked chicken to turn this pasta salad into a complete meal.

# Basil Pesto

Although you can buy pesto in a jar at your local supermarket, nothing compares to the taste and vibrant color of freshly made pesto. It's the perfect condiment to have on hand for sandwiches, pasta, grilled chicken, and other savory dishes.

**MAKES 1 CUP**

**2 cups packed fresh basil**

**½ cup grated Parmesan cheese**

**¼ cup pine nuts**

**3 garlic cloves**

**½ cup extra-virgin olive oil**

Combine the basil, Parmesan cheese, pine nuts, and garlic in a food processor and pulse until well blended. Add the olive oil and pulse again until fully incorporated.

*Cook's note:* Pesto can be stored in a sealed container in the refrigerator for up to 2 weeks.

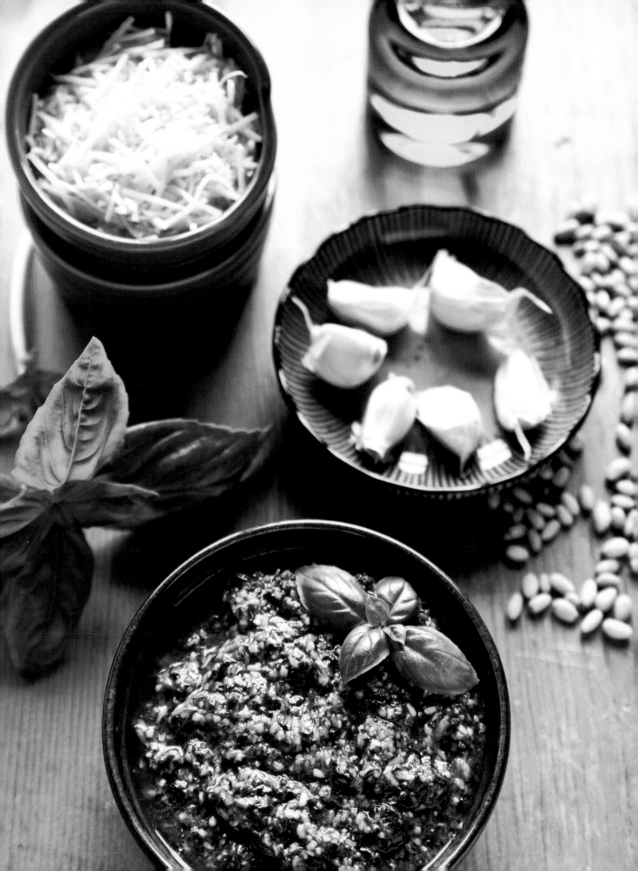

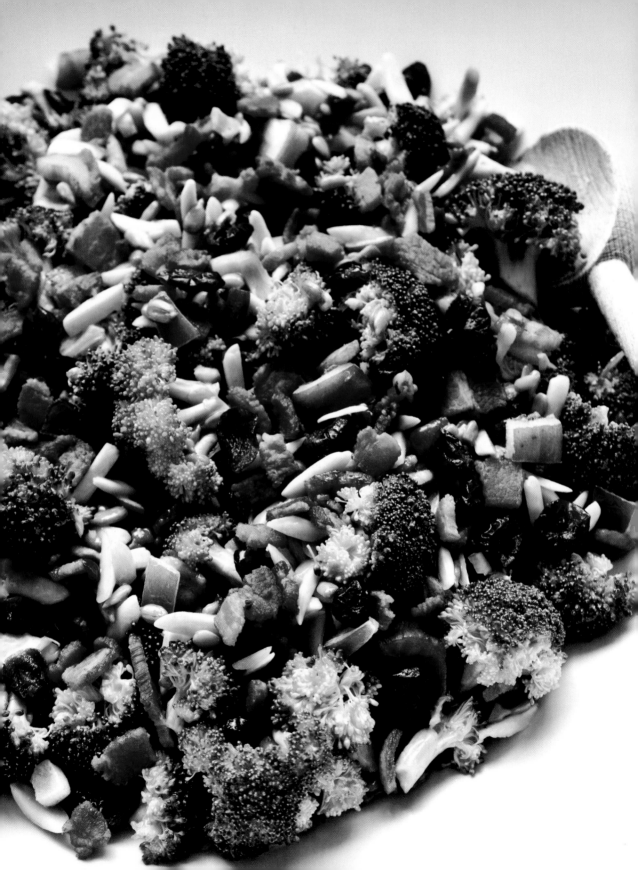

# Broccoli Bacon Salad

Like the perfect black cocktail dress, this classic, nostalgic recipe never goes out of style. The combination of crunchy broccoli and smoky bacon tossed in a sweet and tangy dressing always make this salad popular at potlucks. It's sure to be one of the first dishes to disappear!

1. Combine the broccoli, red onion, cranberries, almonds, and sunflower seeds in a large bowl.

2. To make the dressing, mix the mayonnaise, sugar, vinegar, and pepper together in a small bowl.

3. Pour the dressing over the broccoli salad and mix thoroughly. Transfer the salad to a large plate or serving bowl. Garnish with the crumbled bacon.

*Variation:* If you prefer a vegetarian version, omit the bacon and garnish with another ¼ cup of the cranberries and ¼ cup of the slivered almonds.

*Quality counts:* Good-quality bacon makes the best crumbled bacon bits. Instead of frying whole slices, cut the uncooked bacon into small pieces and then fry them.

*Shopping tip:* If your local grocery store sells ingredients in a bulk bin, you can buy just the amounts of cranberries, almonds, and sunflower seeds you need for this recipe—it's often cheaper and you have no waste afterwards. Most meat departments also sell thick-quality bacon in bulk. Just tell them how much you need.

**SERVES 8 TO 10**

SALAD

**2 fresh broccoli heads, cut into bite-size florets**

**½ cup chopped red onion**

**½ cup dried cranberries**

**½ cup slivered almonds**

**½ cup roasted sunflower seeds**

**1 cup crumbled cooked bacon**

DRESSING

**1 cup mayonnaise**

**⅓ cup granulated sugar**

**3 tablespoons distilled white vinegar**

**½ teaspoon freshly ground black pepper**

# Heavenly Almond Pound Cake

This pound cake is dangerously good. After eating one slice, I often find myself going for seconds . . . then thirds. I love this cake for its velvety texture and the way it melts in your mouth with every bite—heavenly.

**MAKES ONE 10-INCH TUBE CAKE OR TWO 9 x 5 x 3-INCH LOAF CAKES; SERVES 16**

**2 cups (4 sticks) unsalted butter, at room temperature**

**One 8-ounce package cream cheese, at room temperature**

**3 cups granulated sugar**

**6 eggs, at room temperature**

**1 tablespoon almond extract**

**½ teaspoon salt**

**3 cups cake flour**

1. Preheat the oven to 350°F. Generously grease a 10-inch tube pan or two 9 x 5 x 3-inch loaf pans with baking spray.

2. Using a hand or stand mixer, cream the butter, cream cheese, and sugar on medium-high speed for 5 minutes, or until light and fluffy. Beat in the eggs one at a time, then the almond extract and salt. Slowly add the flour and mix for 2 minutes, or until the batter looks smooth. Scrape down the sides and bottom of the bowl and mix for 1 minute more.

3. Pour the cake batter into the tube pan or loaf pans. Using both hands, grab each side of the pan(s) and gently tap the base on the kitchen counter a few times. This helps burst any bubbles caught in the batter, allowing for a tight crumb texture. Bake for 1¼ hours, or until done (see below). Let the cake cool in its pan for 15 minutes.

4. To release the cake from the pan, slowly and carefully run a butter knife along the sides of the pan. Grab each side of the cake pan and gently shake the pan up and down and side to side to loosen the cake; then invert it onto a wire rack to cool. Allow the cake to completely cool before cutting it into clean, beautiful slices.

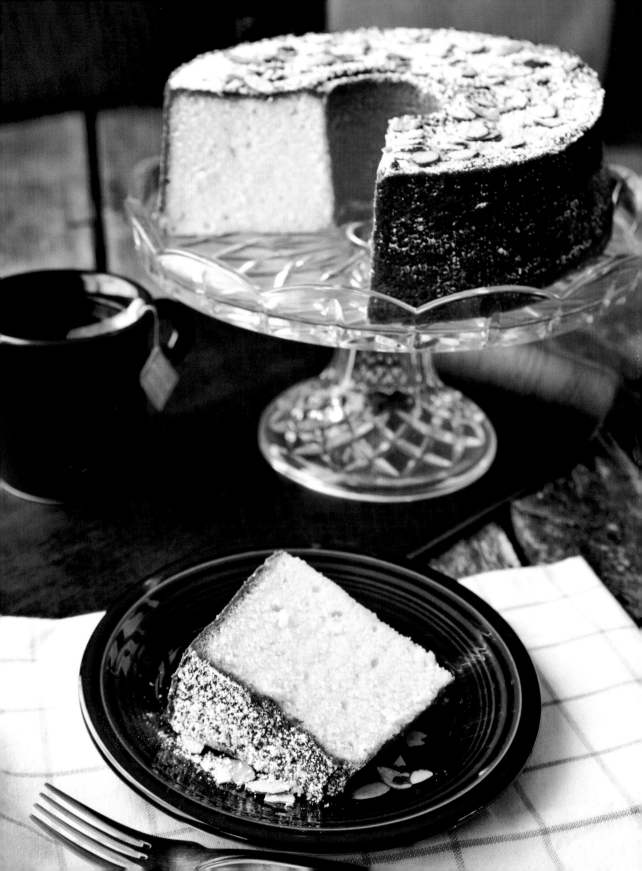

*Testing the cake for doneness:* Stick a wooden skewer into the center of the cake and remove it quickly. If the stick is clean of any cake batter, with only a few crumbs, the cake is completely baked. If any batter is pulled up, bake the cake for 5 minutes longer and test again.

*Avoiding disaster:* Do not let the cake cool in the pan for longer than 15 minutes after removing it from the oven. Otherwise the cake will adhere to the sides of the pan, making it virtually impossible to remove without parts of the cake sticking.

# ten

# DAD'S BIRTHDAY

Celebrating my dad's birthday was never about gifts, balloons, and cards. With every passing year, his only birthday wish was for his children and grandchildren to come together for a family meal. He relished and took pride in his growing family. He would laugh, grinning from ear to ear, whenever someone announced they were expecting a baby, because he loved being a grandpa. The grandkids kept him young in spirit and reminded him that whatever struggles he endured in his life, love does, in fact, conquer all.

Dad lived simply and humbly, and whatever he lacked in material possessions was made up for by the rich blessings of six children and thirteen grandchildren—with two more on the way when he passed. His death was sudden and happened two days after Christmas, while I was writing this book. This chapter is bittersweet for me. What I intended to be a celebration of his favorite foods and a way to honor him is now a dedication to all the birthdays we did celebrate, year after year.

Breaking bread, having fellowship with one another, and giving thanks for the gift of life is what birthdays are about in our family. We're still celebrating Dad on his birthday with his favorite foods as we remember him in photos and stories.

This is dedicated to my dad, who sacrificed so much for us kids so that his ceiling would be our floor. We love and miss you much. I can only imagine the bountiful birthday celebration you must be enjoying each year in heaven.

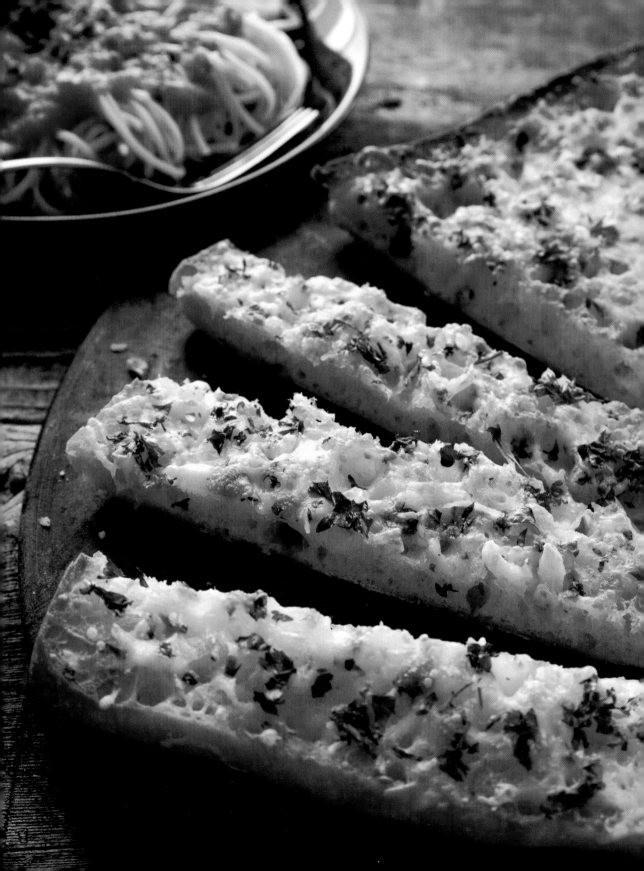

# Garlic Cheese Bread

Who can resist buttery, garlicky, cheesy bread? The aroma wafting from the oven is aromatherapy for the hungry soul. Take one bite of this bread and you'll soon be asking yourself how the heck the whole loaf disappeared so quickly!

1. Preheat the oven to 400°F. Place both halves of the ciabatta bread on a cookie sheet with the cut sides facing up.

2. In a small bowl, combine the butter and garlic until thoroughly mixed. Spread the garlic butter evenly over both halves, making sure to press the garlic butter down with the back of a spatula or knife so the minced garlic is pushed into the air pockets of the bread.

3. Bake the bread for 15 minutes and then remove it from the oven. Change the oven setting to broil. Carefully sprinkle the cheese, then the parsley, over both halves of the bread. Return the bread to the oven and broil for 1 minute, or until the cheese is melted and bubbly.

*Variation:* Consider using Gruyère for a fancier cheese bread.

*Just for fun:* Slice the bread into strips and serve them with a side of warmed marinara sauce for dipping.

**SERVES 8**

1 loaf ciabatta bread, cut in half horizontally

8 tablespoons (1 stick) unsalted butter, at room temperature

4 large garlic cloves, minced

1½ cups shredded cheese of your choice (I like a blend of Parmesan, provolone, and mozzarella)

2 tablespoons finely chopped fresh parsley

# Sautéed Swiss Chard

My father grew Swiss chard in our backyard. He would pick only as many leaves as we needed for that evening's meal, and then Mom would sauté the hearty greens with a little bit of butter, oil, garlic, salt, and pepper. It was the perfect side dish to any meal.

**SERVES 6 TO 8**

2 tablespoons unsalted butter

2 tablespoons extra-virgin olive oil

2 garlic cloves, minced

2 large bunches Swiss chard, stems trimmed, leaves cut crosswise into 1-inch-wide strips

Salt and freshly ground black pepper

Heat the butter and olive oil in a large sauté pan over medium heat until the butter has melted. Add the garlic, then the Swiss chard a few seconds later. Cook the chard, stirring occasionally, until the leaves are tender and wilted, 5 to 7 minutes. Season with salt and pepper.

*Cook's note:* I like to add a squeeze of fresh lemon juice after the Swiss chard has finished cooking. It adds a nice brightness of flavor to this earthy leafy vegetable.

*Variation:* Add a handful of crumbled cooked bacon for an extra dimension of flavor and texture.

*Just for fun:* Use the sautéed Swiss chard and some shredded cheese as a quesadilla filling for a satisfying snack or appetizer.

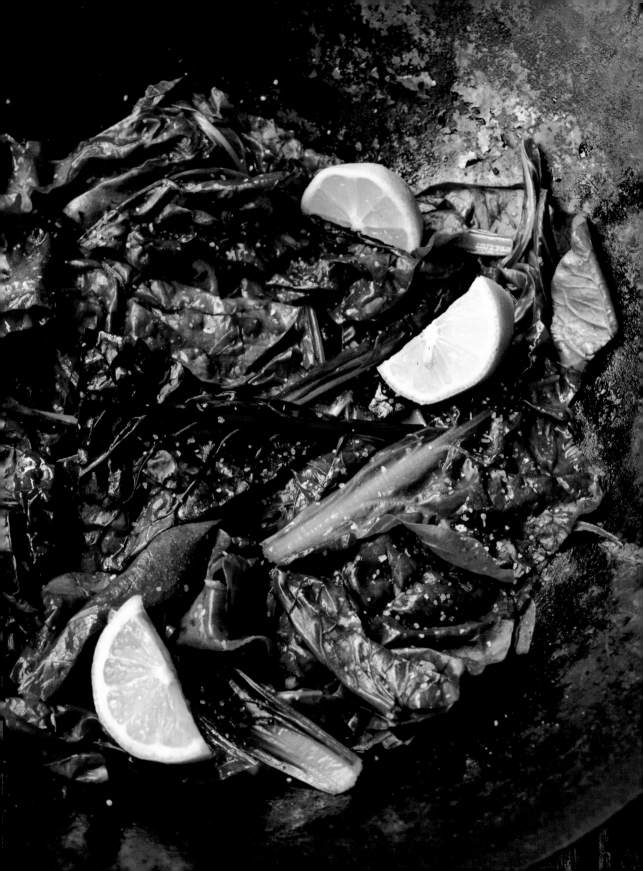

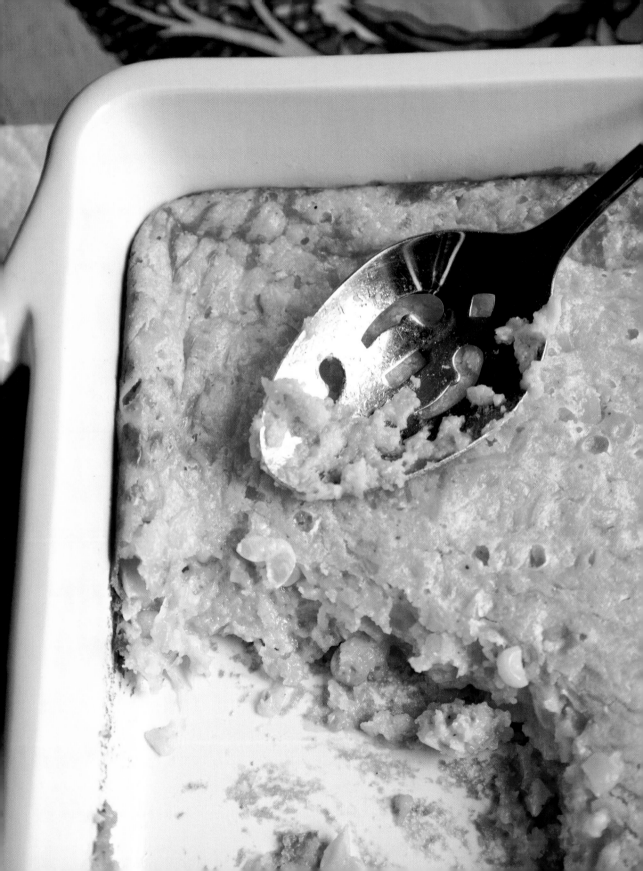

# Corn Pudding

Is it just me or does everyone else get excited when they see corn pudding as part of a special dinner? Personally, I could eat this dish as a main course. The perfect comfort food for the holidays, this corn pudding is a family favorite, and it may well become one of yours too.

1. Preheat the oven to 350°F. Spray a 9 x 13-inch baking dish with nonstick cooking spray.

2. Melt the butter in a large saucepan or Dutch oven over medium heat. Add the onions, garlic, salt, pepper, and cayenne, and sauté for 5 minutes, just until the onions have softened. Turn off the heat.

3. Add the corn kernels, cream-style corn, milk, cream cheese, and sugar, stirring until well combined. Mix in the eggs one at a time, followed by the muffin mix, stirring until the batter is smooth. Stir in the shredded cheese.

4. Pour the mixture into the baking dish and bake for 50 to 60 minutes, until the center is firm.

*Make ahead:* Feel free to make this dish a day in advance and refrigerate it. Then cover the cooked corn pudding with foil, and bake it at 350°F for 20 minutes. You can make the batter, uncooked, a day ahead of time as well—then just follow the normal cooking times.

**SERVES 8**

4 tablespoons (½ stick) unsalted butter

1 small yellow onion, finely chopped

1 large garlic clove, minced

½ teaspoon kosher salt

¼ teaspoon freshly ground black pepper

¼ teaspoon cayenne pepper

2 cups frozen corn kernels, thawed

One 14.5-ounce can cream-style corn

1 cup milk

4 ounces cream cheese, at room temperature

1 tablespoon granulated sugar

2 eggs

One 8.5-ounce box Jiffy corn muffin mix

2 cups shredded sharp cheddar cheese

# Tender Barbecued Ribs

My brother-in-law, Gerald, taught me his secret trick to making tender barbecued ribs—the meat practically falls off the bones. His method of preboiling them before finishing them off on the grill is genius and results in some of the best ribs our family has ever tasted.

**SERVES 4 TO 6**

**4 pounds baby back pork ribs**

**3 tablespoons kosher salt**

**3 cups store-bought barbecue sauce (I love Sweet Baby Ray's)**

1. Place the ribs and salt in a large heavy pot and add water to cover. Bring to a boil over medium-high heat. Then reduce the heat to medium-low and simmer for 45 minutes. Using tongs, carefully remove the ribs from the pot and set them aside on a baking sheet to cool slightly. Cut the ribs into smaller, individual sections (4 to 6 ribs each) or into individual pieces.

2. Heat an outdoor grill to medium-high. Brush barbecue sauce thickly on both sides of the ribs. Grill each side for 3 minutes. Repeat this process of basting and grilling 2 more times. The ribs are now ready to be devoured!

*Time-saving tip:* Cook the ribs in a pressure cooker for 20 minutes instead of boiling them on the stovetop. This method produces the tenderest barbecued ribs in under an hour. Gotta love that!

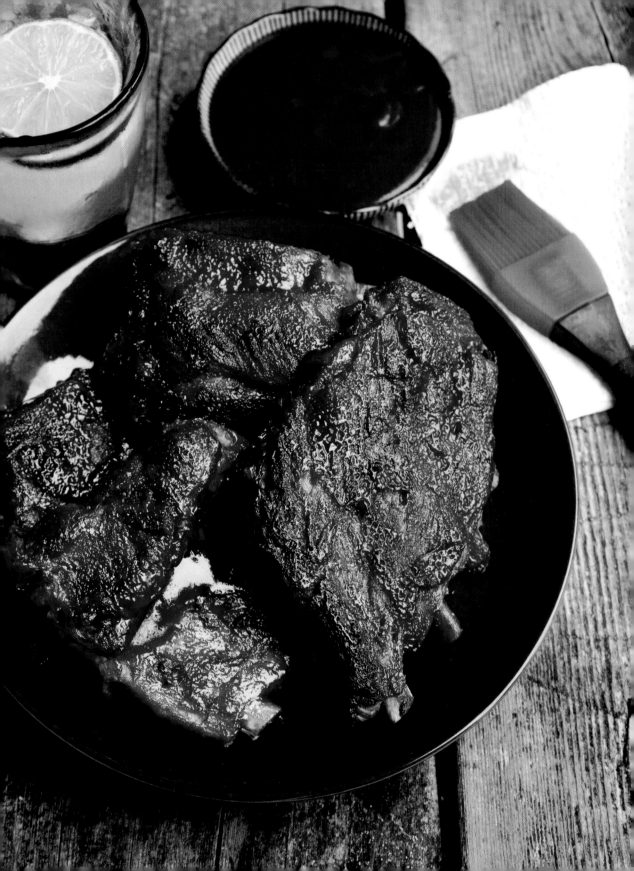

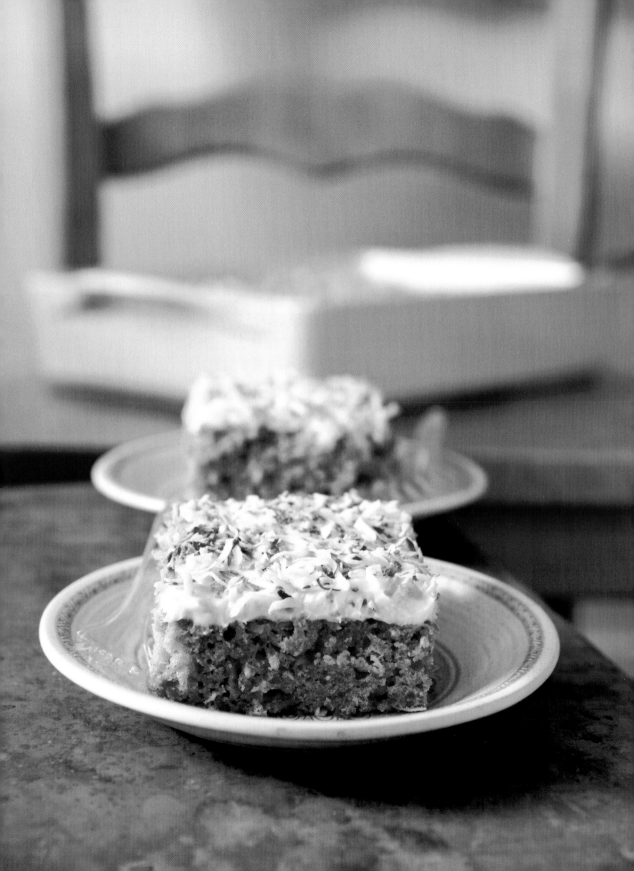

# Dad's Carrot Cake

Carrot cake recipes vary in taste, texture, and frosting—and people are apt to have strong preferences. I perfected this recipe for my dad, who liked his cake light and moist with just a hint of spice. Top it off with a fluffy cream cheese frosting—the perfect complement!

1. Preheat the oven to 350°F. Spray a 9 x 13-inch baking dish with nonstick cooking spray.

2. Using a hand or stand mixer, mix the eggs, oil, applesauce, and vanilla extract on low speed for 30 seconds. Beat in both sugars on medium speed until well combined, 2 minutes. Add the flour, baking powder, cinnamon, salt, and nutmeg. Mix the batter until the dry ingredients are fully incorporated. Stir in the carrots on low speed until they are evenly distributed within the batter. Pour the batter into the baking dish and spread it evenly with a spatula.

3. Bake for 40 to 45 minutes, until the center of the cake springs back when touched. Allow the cake to cool completely in its pan before topping it with the Whipped Cream Cheese Frosting. If you like, sprinkle the frosted cake with toasted coconut. Cut into squares to serve.

*Cook's Note:* This cake tastes better if you prepare it a day in advance and refrigerate it overnight, giving the cake time to set up and allowing the texture to come together.

**SERVES 12**

4 eggs

½ cup vegetable oil

½ cup applesauce

2 teaspoons pure vanilla extract

1 cup granulated sugar

1 cup firmly packed dark brown sugar

2 cups all-purpose flour

1 tablespoon baking powder

1 teaspoon ground cinnamon

½ teaspoon salt

¼ teaspoon ground nutmeg

4 cups grated carrots

Whipped Cream Cheese Frosting (recipe follows)

1 cup toasted sweetened coconut (optional)

# Whipped Cream Cheese Frosting

**MAKES 2 CUPS**

**One 8-ounce package cream cheese, at room temperature**

**1 cup confectioners' sugar, sifted**

**½ cup heavy cream**

Using a hand or stand mixer, whip all the ingredients together on low speed until the sugar is fully absorbed. Increase the speed to medium-high and blend until the mixture resembles frosting. Don't worry if the mixture initially looks curdled. Keep whipping it and watch it transform into a thick frosting.

# eleven

# GAME DAY

Like many American women, I've learned a thing or two when it comes to men and college football. When game day arrives I stop being the focus of my husband's attention. I become invisible as Rob channels all his energy toward the big screen, watching his beloved Washington State Cougars with friends or by himself.

Seeing him delight in a game is like watching the sheer happiness our kids get from their favorite movies, so I don't mind giving him the afternoon off—that is, unless it's the Apple Cup rivalry and the University of Washington Huskies are playing. In that case, I join Rob on the couch and engage in obnoxious trash talking that's unbecoming of a mother of three. "Go Huskies, go Huskies!" I scream as I do the running man dance, followed by something akin to MC Hammer's moves in his "Can't Touch This" video. I have no shame, and no coordination whatsoever. But I can tell you this: We have a lot of fun teasing each other while munching on our favorite game-day food. Whoever wins or loses, game days are always a blast at our house, and the food is a big part of the enjoyment.

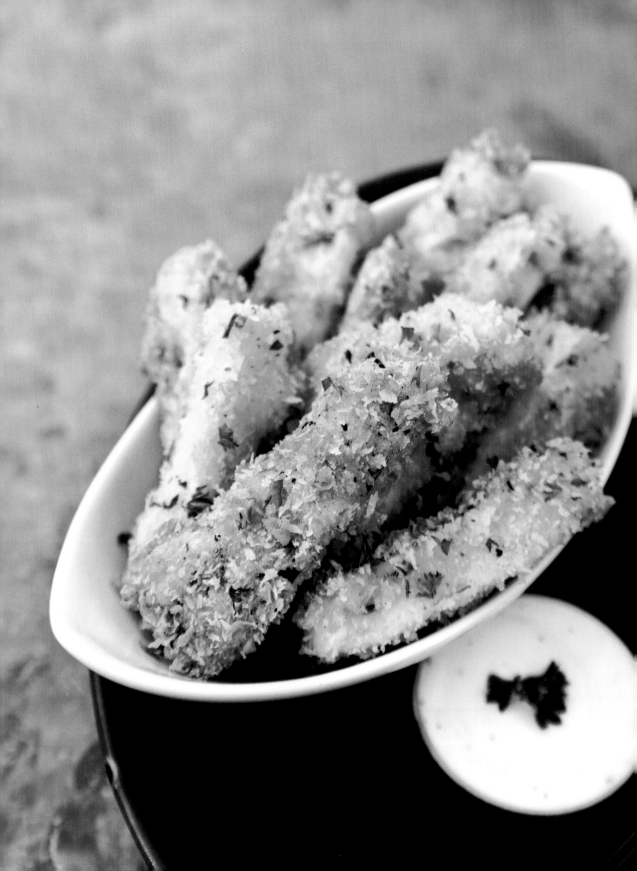

# Deep-Fried Zucchini Sticks

Deep-fried zucchini sticks are one of my most favorite foods in the world! They're typically served as an appetizer, but I could eat a whole plate of them as a main dish. Pair these with ranch dressing for dipping and you have a winning combination.

1. In a heavy pot or a deep fryer, heat 2 inches of vegetable or peanut oil to 350°F.

2. In a shallow bowl, combine the flour, garlic salt, and pepper. Pour the beaten eggs into a separate bowl. In a third dish, combine the panko breadcrumbs and the Parmesan cheese.

3. Dredge the zucchini sticks in the flour, followed by the egg, and finally the panko-cheese mixture. Lay the breaded zucchini sticks on a baking sheet as you finish coating them.

4. Working in small batches, deep-fry the zucchini until golden brown, about 30 seconds. Carefully remove the zucchini from the hot oil and drain on a plate lined with paper towels. Sprinkle with the fresh parsley and serve with a side of ranch dressing.

*Like it spicy?* Mix 2 teaspoons cayenne pepper into the panko-Parmesan mixture for a little heat.

**SERVES 6**

Vegetable or peanut oil, for frying

½ cup all-purpose flour

1 tablespoon garlic salt

1 teaspoon freshly ground black pepper

3 eggs, beaten

1½ cups panko breadcrumbs

1 cup grated Parmesan cheese

3 medium zucchini, cut crosswise into 3-inch segments, each segment quartered lengthwise

2 tablespoons chopped fresh parsley

Ranch dressing, for serving

# Caramelized Onion Clam Dip

If I had to confess to a guilty pleasure, it would be snacking on this dip with my favorite thick-cut ruffled potato chips. Sometimes I even sneak a spoonful of it when no one is looking. I created this dip for my husband and me to indulge in when we're up late studying or blogging, and it has become one of our favorite late-night and game-day treats.

**MAKES 3 CUPS**

2 tablespoons unsalted butter

1 medium yellow onion, chopped

1½ teaspoons dried thyme

1½ teaspoons garlic salt

1½ teaspoons granulated sugar

¼ teaspoon cayenne pepper

¼ teaspoon freshly ground black pepper

One 8-ounce can minced clams, drained, juices reserved

½ cup sour cream

One 8-ounce package cream cheese, at room temperature

½ teaspoon liquid smoke

Potato chips, for serving

1. In a medium skillet over medium heat, melt the butter. Add the onions, thyme, garlic salt, sugar, cayenne, and black pepper. Stirring occasionally, cook the onions for 10 minutes, or until soft and nicely browned. Add the clam juice and simmer until the liquid has reduced by half. Remove the skillet from the heat and set aside to cool.

2. In a medium bowl, mix the sour cream, cream cheese, and liquid smoke until well combined. Add the cooled onion mixture and the minced clams, and stir until all the ingredients are fully incorporated. Serve with your favorite potato chips.

*Cook's note:* Liquid smoke is a seasoning that adds a smoky flavor to foods. It can be found in the condiment section of most grocery stores.

*Make ahead:* This dip can be made up to 2 days in advance. Just be sure to keep it covered and refrigerated until ready to use.

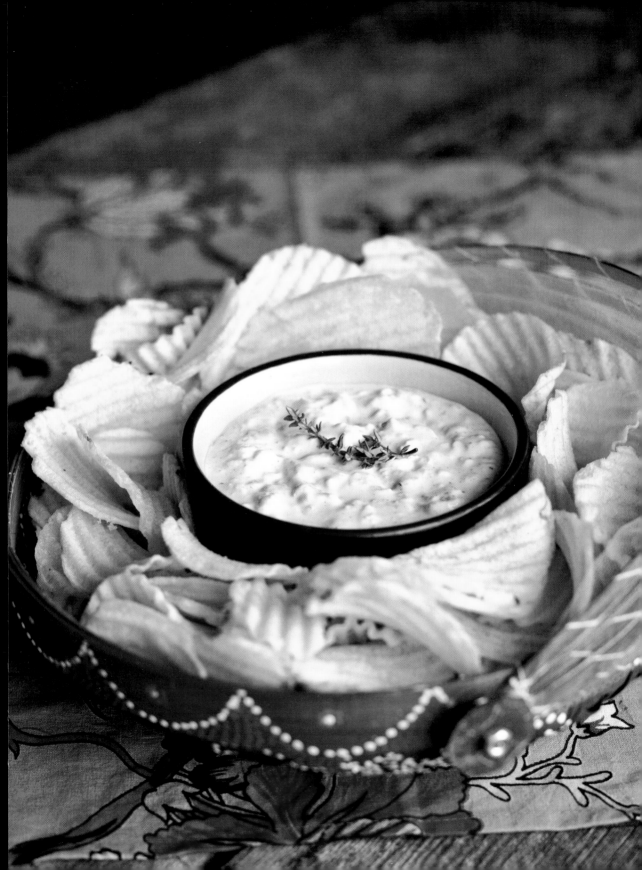

# Game-Day Steak Nachos

Give my husband a platter of nachos and he heads straight for the couch. With a TV remote in one hand and a nice cold beer in the other, it can mean only one thing: it's time to watch some football. These game-day nachos are perfect for snacking while cheering your favorite team on to victory.

**SERVES 8**

3 tablespoons extra-virgin olive oil

1 pound boneless top sirloin steak

Kosher salt and freshly ground black pepper

One 15-ounce can black beans

½ teaspoon ground cumin

One 18-ounce bag corn tortilla chips

2 cups shredded cheddar cheese

One 2.25-ounce can sliced black olives, drained

2 green onions, thinly sliced (use green and white parts)

2 Roma tomatoes, chopped

¼ cup chopped fresh cilantro

Sour cream

1. Preheat the oven to 350°F. Place a large skillet over medium-high heat.

2. Rub 1 tablespoon of the olive oil on both sides of the steak, and season the steak generously with salt and pepper. Add the remaining 2 tablespoons oil to the skillet, and cook the steak for 5 minutes on each side for medium-rare. Remove the steak from the skillet and transfer it to a cutting board. Allow the steak to rest for 5 minutes.

3. While the steak is resting, prepare the black beans: Pour the beans into a strainer and rinse them. Place the beans and the cumin in a medium saucepan, and heat over medium heat for 5 minutes, or until warmed through.

4. Cut the steak into ⅓-inch cubes.

5. Layer the tortilla chips on a large baking sheet, sprinkling cheese between the layers of chips. Sprinkle the chips with a top layer of cheese, and then with the steak bits, black beans, olives, and green onions. Bake for 10 minutes, or until the cheese has melted.

6. Scatter the tomatoes and cilantro over the nachos. Spoon a big dollop of sour cream on top, and serve immediately.

*Other great toppings to consider:* pepper Jack cheese, chopped red onion, sliced jalapeños, peperoncini slices, shredded chicken, guacamole, salsa.

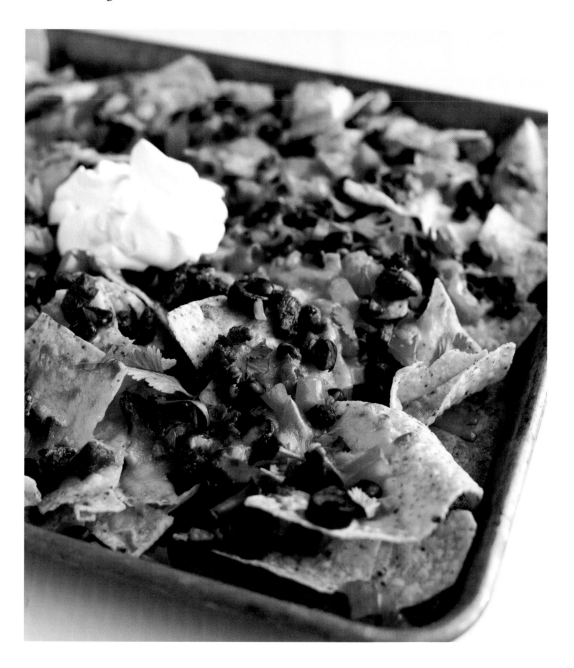

# Sweet and Spicy Wings

They say the way to a man's heart is through his stomach. The way to my man's heart is through these sweet and spicy wings. When a big game is on TV, I make a special batch just for Rob. Double-frying the wings and tossing them in an Asian-inspired sauce elevates these chicken wings from ordinary to extraordinary.

**SERVES 4 TO 6**

**3 pounds chicken wings, each separated into 2 pieces, wing tips removed and discarded**

**Salt and freshly ground black pepper**

**½ cup whole milk**

SWEET AND SPICY SAUCE

**⅓ cup honey**

**¼ cup granulated sugar**

**3 tablespoons soy sauce**

**2 tablespoons rice vinegar**

**3 large garlic cloves, chopped**

**1 tablespoon Asian sesame oil**

**2 teaspoons minced fresh ginger**

**1 teaspoon cayenne pepper**

**Peanut oil, for frying**

**1 cup cornstarch**

**2 tablespoons toasted sesame seeds**

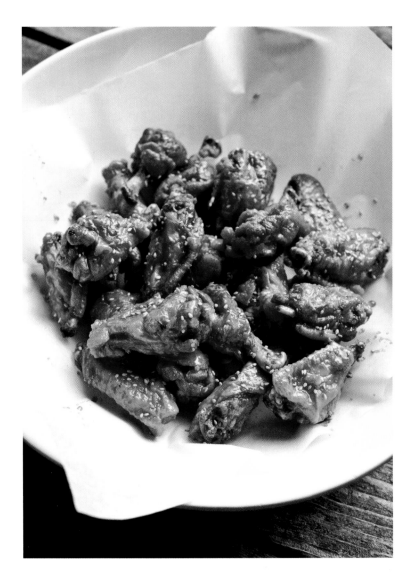

1. Lay the chicken wing parts in a 9 x 13-inch baking dish and season them generously with salt and pepper. Add the milk, and marinate the chicken for 20 minutes.

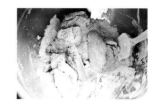

2. Meanwhile, make the sweet and spicy sauce: Whisk the honey, sugar, soy sauce, rice vinegar, garlic, sesame oil, ginger, and cayenne together in a medium saucepan. Bring the sauce to a boil over medium-high heat, and cook for 1 minute. Then reduce the heat to low and simmer for 5 minutes. Turn off the heat and set the sauce aside to cool.

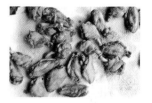

3. Pour 3 inches of peanut oil into a heavy pot and heat the oil to 350°F over medium-high heat. When the oil is nearly ready, dredge half the chicken wings in the cornstarch. Fry the wings in the hot oil for 5 minutes. Transfer the cooked wings to a plate lined with paper towels. Dredge and fry the second batch of wings. Then fry each batch again for 5 minutes, or until golden brown.

4. When all the wings have been fried for a second time, transfer them to a large heatproof bowl. Pour the sweet and spicy sauce over the wings, and turn them with a spatula until they are completely coated in sauce. Transfer the wings to a serving plate and sprinkle them with toasted sesame seeds.

*Butcher's tip:* Most grocery store butchers will cut the wings into two pieces for you, removing and discarding the tips, if you ask them *nicely*.

# Chocolate Cupcakes with Peanut Butter Cookie Frosting

I am a self-proclaimed cupcake connoisseur. In order for a cupcake to pass my stringent test of excellence, it must meet the following criteria: First and foremost, the cupcake must be beautiful—visual appeal is the primary factor in determining whether or not I'll want to eat it. Bonus points are awarded for creativity. Once the cupcake passes the cuteness test, it also needs to taste as good as it looks. The cake should be moist and the frosting should complement the cake flavor and texture. Here I present to you one of my all-time favorite cupcakes. They're topped off with two different frostings: a rich, decadent ganache and a salty-sweet peanut butter cookie frosting. The chocolate–peanut butter combination is to die for, rightfully earning this cupcake five stars in my book.

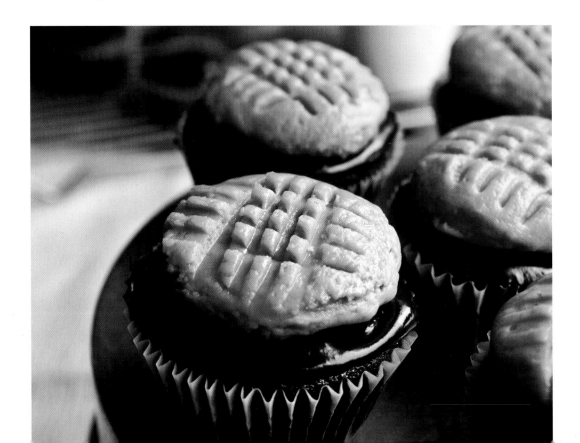

1. Preheat the oven to 350°F. Line 1 or 2 muffin tins with 18 paper liners.

2. In a small bowl, whisk the coffee and cocoa powder together until the mixture resembles a smooth chocolate sauce; set aside to cool.

3. Using a hand or stand mixer, cream the butter and both sugars together on medium speed until fluffy, about 3 minutes. Add the eggs one at a time, beating well after each addition. Then add the vanilla extract. Slowly add the flour, baking soda, baking powder, and salt, and mix on low speed for 2 minutes. Add the chocolate-coffee mixture, and mix the batter for 1 minute more. Scrape down the bottom and sides of the bowl, and mix on medium-high speed for 2 minutes, or until the batter is smooth.

4. Fill each muffin cup about two-thirds full. Bake for 25 minutes, or until the center of a cupcake springs back when touched.

5. While the cupcakes are baking, prepare the ganache glaze and the peanut butter cookie frosting. To make the ganache, heat the heavy cream in a small pot over medium-high heat. As soon as the cream begins to boil, remove the pot from the heat and add the chocolate chips. Stir together with a whisk until smooth. Pour the ganache into a medium bowl and cool it in the refrigerator while the cupcakes are baking.

6. To make the peanut butter cookie frosting, cream the peanut butter and butter together for 1 minute on medium speed. Turn off the mixer and add the confectioners' sugar. Beat the frosting on low speed until all the sugar has been absorbed.

MAKES 18
CUPCAKES

CUPCAKES

1 cup strong hot brewed coffee

½ cup unsweetened cocoa powder

8 tablespoons (1 stick) unsalted butter, at room temperature

1 cup firmly packed dark brown sugar

½ cup granulated sugar

2 eggs

1½ teaspoons pure vanilla extract

1½ cups all-purpose flour

1 teaspoon baking soda

½ teaspoon baking powder

¼ teaspoon salt

CHOCOLATE GANACHE

½ cup heavy cream

1 cup semisweet chocolate chips

PEANUT BUTTER COOKIE FROSTING

1 cup creamy peanut butter (I use Skippy Natural Creamy)

6 tablespoons (¾ stick) unsalted butter, at room temperature

2 cups confectioners' sugar, sifted

Then increase the speed to medium and mix the frosting for 2 minutes. Cover and refrigerate until ready to use.

**7.** Transfer the cupcakes to a wire rack and let them cool completely.

**8.** When the cupcakes are completely cooled, spoon 1 tablespoon of the ganache glaze on top of each cupcake. Using the back of a spoon, spread the ganache evenly over the entire surface. Allow the ganache to set for 30 minutes.

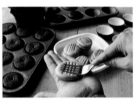

**9.** While the ganache is setting, use clean, dry hands to form eighteen 1-tablespoon balls of the peanut butter frosting, rolling each ball between your palms until the surface is smooth. (Each ball should be slightly smaller than a Ping-Pong ball. The frosting ball should easily keep its shape without sticking to anything.) With both hands, gently squish each frosting ball to form a ⅓-inch-thick patty. Using the tines of a fork, indent the top of the patty in a crisscross pattern so that it resembles a peanut butter cookie.

**10.** Place a frosting "cookie" on top of each cupcake.

# twelve

# WELCOME HOME

As fun as it is to eat out once in a while, it can get old very quickly if you have to travel often. For two years, Rob traveled around the country every other week for work. Each night we talked on the phone and recapped our day, and I often asked him what he ate for dinner. I would live vicariously through him as he described in detail every little bite he had. To me it seemed so glamorous, but to him (and to my surprise), nothing could beat a home-cooked meal.

It wasn't until I started to travel myself that I understood what he meant. Nothing can substitute for family gathered around a table eating a lovingly prepared meal—this experience can't be ordered off a menu.

Now when Rob comes home from a business trip, I make an earnest effort to bless him by tidying up the house and making sure I have a home-cooked meal waiting for him the moment he walks through the door. By the time we all sit down for dinner, I make it a point to watch him throughout the meal. It brings me great pleasure to see him enjoy every bite. After all, there's no place like home.

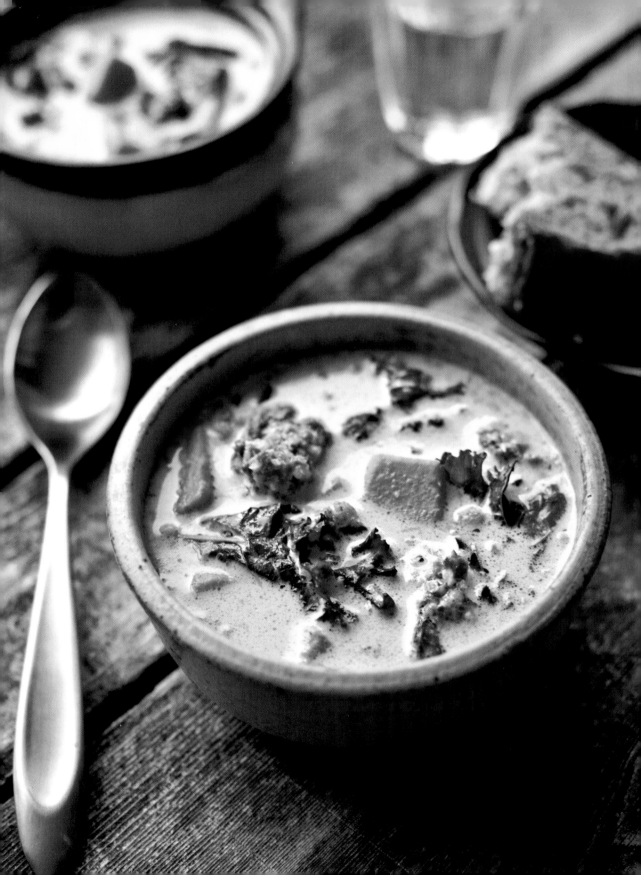

# Spicy Sausage Kale Bean Soup

This soup is perfect for a cold winter night, especially when I need dinner on the table rather quickly but want something that tastes delicious. It can be ready in less than 30 minutes and needs only a side of warm rustic bread to complete the meal.

1. In a large Dutch oven or soup pot over medium heat, cook the sausage, onion, and garlic for 5 minutes, or until the onion has softened and the sausage is browned. Remove any excess fat drippings.

2. Add the chicken broth, cream, cannellini beans, and sweet potatoes. Cover the pot and bring the soup to a boil. Then reduce the heat to low and simmer for 15 minutes.

3. Stir in the kale and cook for 5 more minutes, still covered. Serve each bowl of soup with a slice of rustic bread.

*Too spicy?* Substitute mild sweet Italian pork sausage for the hot Italian pork sausage.

**SERVES 6 TO 8**

1 pound hot Italian pork sausage meat, crumbled

½ medium onion, chopped

3 garlic cloves, chopped

One 32-ounce carton chicken broth

2 cups heavy cream

One 14-ounce can cannellini beans, rinsed and drained

2 sweet potatoes, peeled and cubed

1 bunch kale, coarsely chopped

Rustic bread, for serving

# Pear Gorgonzola Pecan Salad

This is my favorite fall and winter salad. I love how the maple pecan vinaigrette enhances the flavor of each ingredient. The natural sweetness of the pears, the creaminess of the Gorgonzola, and the crunch of the candied pecans complement one another for an incredible salad.

**SERVES 4 TO 6**

**5 to 6 cups mixed field greens**

**2 firm but ripe Bartlett pears, cored and thinly sliced**

**1 cup crumbled Gorgonzola cheese**

**1 cup Candied Pecans (page 217), chopped**

**Maple Pecan Vinaigrette (recipe follows)**

In a large serving bowl, toss the greens, pears, cheese, and pecans. Drizzle with the vinaigrette, and toss again.

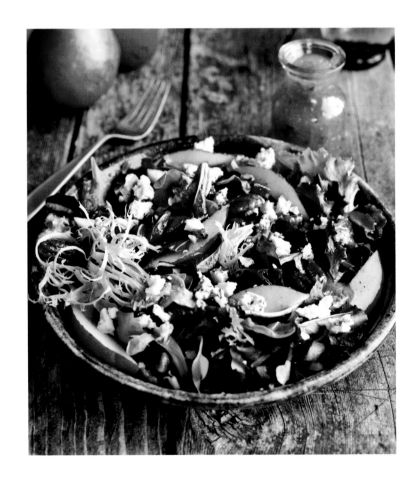

# Maple Pecan Vinaigrette

Combine the olive oil, vinegar, maple syrup, pecans, and cayenne in a food processor or blender, and blend for 10 seconds. (If you don't have a food processor or blender, you can whisk the vinaigrette ingredients. Just be sure to crush the pecans with a rolling pin first to get them as fine as possible.)

*Cook's note:* I like to make a double batch of this vinaigrette to use again later. It can be stored in the refrigerator for up to a month.

**MAKES ¾ CUP**

¼ cup extra-virgin olive oil

3 tablespoons apple cider vinegar

3 tablespoons pure maple syrup

12 Candied Pecans (page 217)

¼ teaspoon cayenne pepper

# Acorn Squash with Brown Sugar Butter Sauce

Acorn squash is one of my favorite side dishes during the fall and winter months. The spiced brown sugar butter sauce adds just enough sweetness to it without being overpowering. My method for preparing this dish takes less than half the time typically required to bake the squash in the oven, and without compromising texture or flavor. It's simply perfect.

**SERVES 2 TO 4**

1 acorn squash, halved, stringy pulp and seeds removed

4 tablespoons (½ stick) unsalted butter, melted

2 tablespoons honey

6 tablespoons firmly packed dark brown sugar

1 teaspoon ground cinnamon

½ teaspoon ground nutmeg

¼ teaspoon kosher salt

1. Pour ½ cup water into a microwave-safe casserole that is large enough to accommodate both squash pieces. Place the squash flesh-side down in the dish and microwave for 15 minutes, or until the squash is tender.

2. While the squash is cooking, whisk the butter, honey, brown sugar, cinnamon, nutmeg, and salt in a small bowl and set aside.

3. Preheat the broiler.

4. Transfer the squash to a baking sheet, flesh-side up. (Be careful—it will be very hot.) Generously brush the rim and inside surface of each piece with the brown sugar mixture. Divide any remaining sauce between the 2 pieces, pouring it into the scooped-out center. Broil for 2 to 3 minutes, or until the edges of the squash have caramelized.

*Just for fun:* Sprinkle a little bit of brown sugar on the edges of the squash before broiling to achieve a more oven-caramelized look.

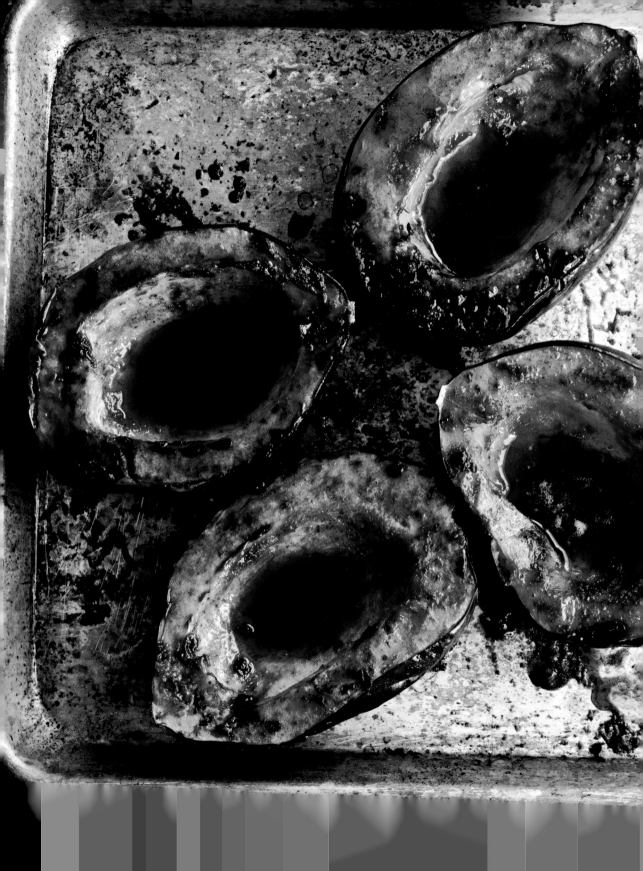

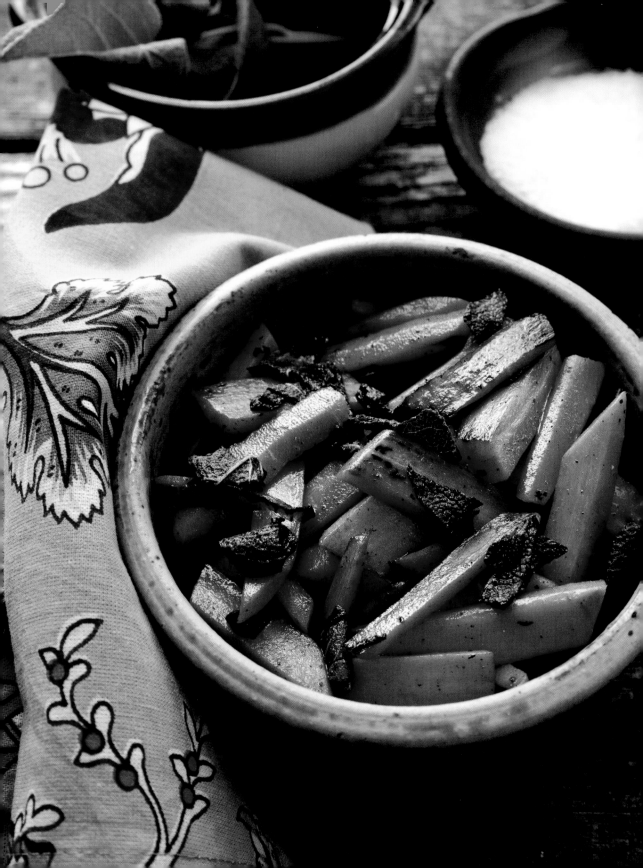

# Roasted Carrots with Sage Brown Butter

I'll never forget Abbi and Mimi's reaction when I asked them to try eating crispy sage leaves cooked in brown butter. They were scared out of their minds . . . until they took their first bite. Then they asked me to make more! Adding the sage brown butter to roasted carrots gives them a unique flavor that I absolutely love—and the kids love too!

1. Preheat the oven to 400°F.

2. In a large bowl, toss the carrots with the olive oil to coat them thoroughly. Spread the carrots in a single layer on a baking sheet and roast them for 20 minutes, or until tender.

3. Meanwhile, prepare the sage brown butter: Melt the butter in a small saucepan over medium heat. Add the sage, cinnamon, and nutmeg and cook until the butter is fragrant, brown, and beginning to foam, 1 to 2 minutes. Remove the pan from the heat and set aside.

4. Toss the carrots in the sage brown butter and season them with salt and pepper to taste before serving.

*Just for fun:* Sprinkle a little bit of brown sugar on the carrots right before you roast them. The added sugar brings out the natural sweetness of the carrots, which complements the nuttiness of the brown butter.

**SERVES 6**

12 carrots, peeled, cut in half lengthwise, then cut into 2-inch pieces

2 tablespoons extra-virgin olive oil

3 tablespoons salted butter

6 fresh sage leaves, chopped

¼ teaspoon ground cinnamon

¼ teaspoon ground nutmeg

Kosher salt and freshly ground black pepper

# Scalloped Potato Leek Gratin

If you ask me, potatoes and cheese were destined to be together, like peanut butter and jelly. This comfort dish goes well with just about everything. It can be served for breakfast, brunch, or dinner and is fancy enough to include on your holiday menu.

**SERVES 6 TO 8**

2 large leeks, trimmed and halved lengthwise (use green and white parts)

2 tablespoons salted butter

Kosher salt and freshly ground black pepper

1½ cups heavy cream

2 garlic cloves, chopped

½ teaspoon ground nutmeg

½ teaspoon dried thyme

2 pounds Yukon Gold or russet potatoes, unpeeled, sliced ⅛-inch thick

½ cup shredded cheddar cheese

⅓ cup grated Parmesan cheese

1. Preheat the oven to 375°F. Spray a medium casserole dish with nonstick cooking spray.

2. Wash the leeks, removing any grit. Thinly slice the leeks crosswise. In a large skillet, melt the butter over medium heat. Add the leeks, ½ teaspoon kosher salt, and ¼ teaspoon pepper. Cook until the leeks are tender, about 5 minutes. Transfer the leeks to a bowl. Add the cream, garlic, nutmeg, and thyme to the skillet. Cook the cream mixture over medium heat for 5 minutes, stirring occasionally. Remove the cream sauce from the heat.

3. Place a layer of potato slices in an overlapping pattern in the casserole dish, seasoning the potatoes with a little salt and pepper. Scatter all the leeks over the potatoes, followed by a third of the cream sauce and then a third of cheese. Repeat the layers of potatoes, sauce, and cheese 2 more times. Bake the gratin, uncovered, for 50 minutes, or until the cheese is bubbly and golden.

*Cook's note:* If you plan on doubling the recipe, the baking time should be doubled as well.

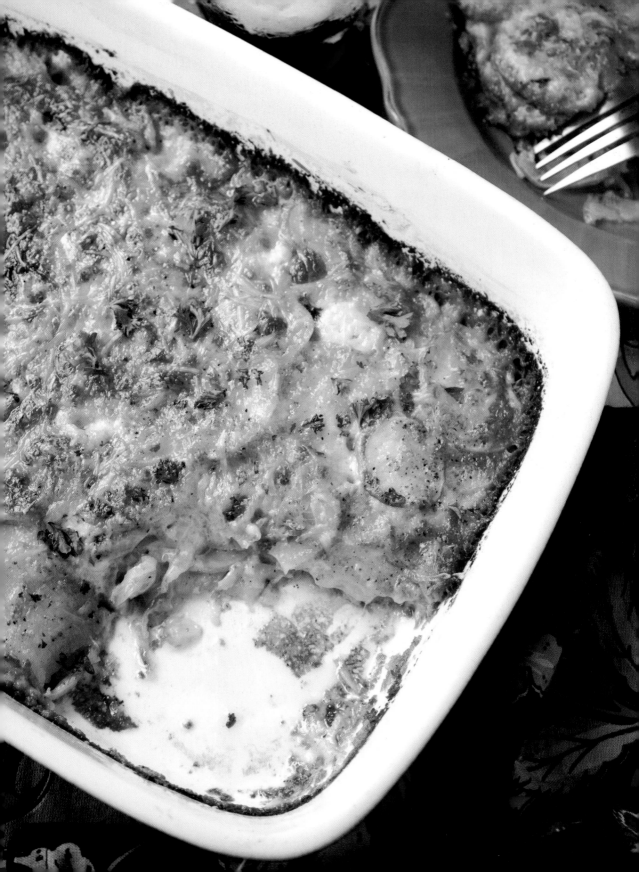

# Pork Chops with Apple Chutney

My husband's multiethnic (East Indian/Pakistani and European American) background is the inspiration behind this recipe. He loves it when I serve pork chops for dinner, but his face really lights up when I surprise him by adding this sweet and spiced apple chutney to go with them.

**SERVES 6**

1 Granny Smith apple, peeled, cored, and chopped

1 sweet apple (such as Braeburn or Fuji), peeled, cored, and chopped

½ cup firmly packed dark brown sugar

¼ cup apple cider vinegar

¼ cup orange juice

¼ cup raisins

½ teaspoon minced fresh ginger

½ teaspoon cornstarch

½ teaspoon ground cinnamon

¼ teaspoon ground cloves

Six 1-inch-thick boneless pork loin chops

Kosher salt and freshly ground black pepper

¾ cup all-purpose flour

¼ cup extra-virgin olive oil

1. First, start the apple chutney: Combine the apples, brown sugar, cider vinegar, orange juice, raisins, ginger, cornstarch, cinnamon, and cloves in a medium pot, and bring to a boil over medium heat. Reduce the heat to a low simmer, and simmer for 10 minutes, or until the apples are cooked through and the liquid has reduced to a thick syrup.

2. Meanwhile, prepare the pork chops: Generously season both sides of the pork chops with salt and pepper. Dredge both sides of the pork chops in the flour, and shake off any excess. Heat the oil in a large skillet over medium-high heat. Place the pork chops in the skillet, taking care not to overcrowd them, and cook for 5 minutes on each side, or until golden brown and cooked through. (If necessary, pan-fry the pork chops in batches, adding more oil if needed.) Transfer the pork chops to individual plates and top with the chutney.

*How to check pork for doneness:* Make a small cut into the center of the chop, about ¼ to ½ inch deep. The pork is done when the center is white. If the juice from the meat is not clear, or is still slightly pink, the pork chops should be returned to the pan for further cooking.

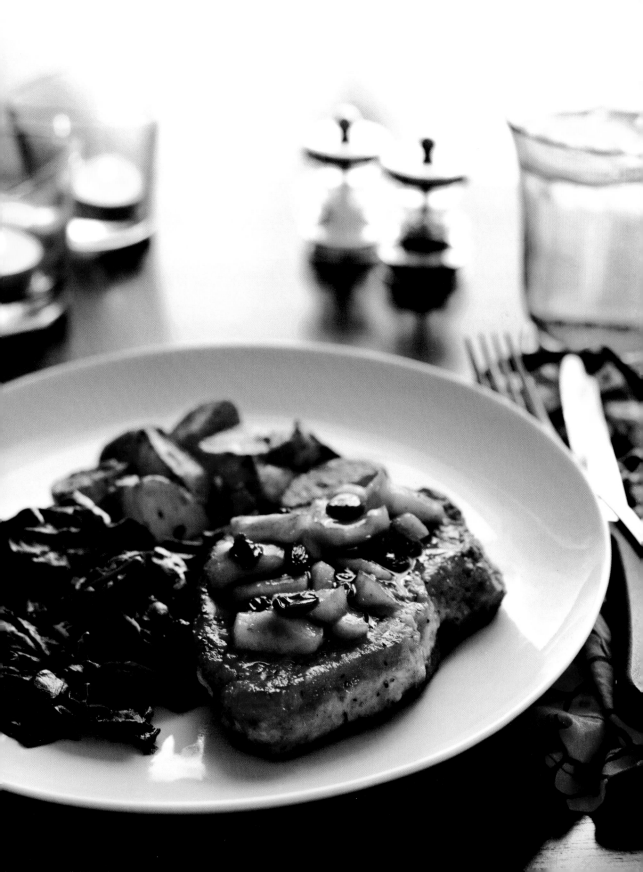

# Rustic Spiced Plum Tart

I love the simplicity of this dessert. It is so easy to prepare and never fails to impress every time I make it for friends and family.

**One 9-inch unbaked pie crust (store-bought or homemade)**

**¼ cup crushed cinnamon graham crackers**

**1 pound red plums, pitted and cut into ¼-inch-thick slices**

**½ cup granulated sugar**

**1 tablespoon all-purpose flour**

**½ teaspoon ground cardamom**

**¼ teaspoon ground cinnamon**

**Egg wash: 1 egg yolk mixed with 1 teaspoon water**

**2 tablespoons raw sugar**

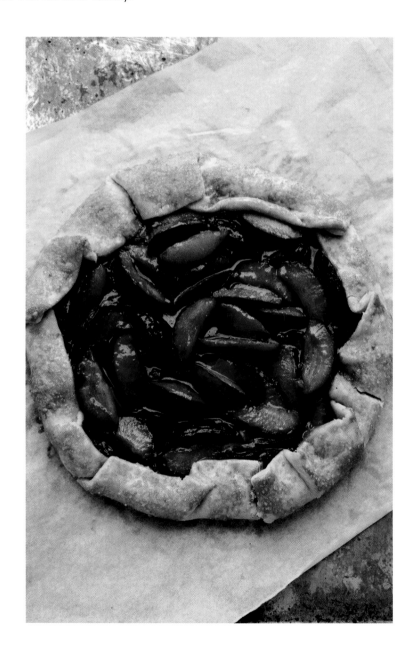

1. Preheat the oven to 400°F. Line a baking sheet with parchment paper.

2. Lay the pie crust flat on top of the parchment paper. Spread the graham cracker crumbs over the center of the crust, leaving a 2-inch border around the edges.

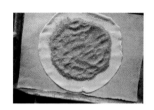

3. In a large bowl, toss the plums, sugar, flour, cardamom, and cinnamon together to coat the plums thoroughly. Mound the plums on top of the crumbs.

4. Fold the edges of the crust over the fruit, pleating the dough as you go and leaving the center exposed. Brush the outside edges with the egg wash, and sprinkle the raw sugar around the border. Bake for 45 minutes, or until the crust is golden and the filling is bubbling.

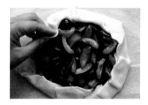

*Cook's note:* Don't be concerned if some of the juices from the filling spill over. This is normal and adds to the rustic look.

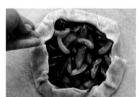

*Just for fun:* Serve each slice with a scoop of vanilla or ginger ice cream to elevate this tart to a fancy and memorable dessert!

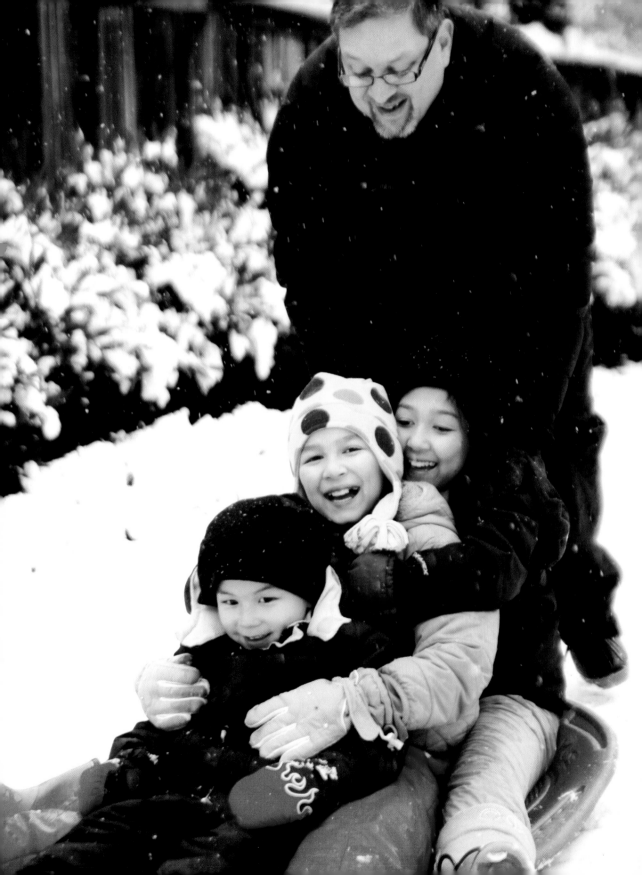

# thirteen

# SNOW DAY

Waking up to snow flurries outside my window always gives me a sense of childlike excitement. When the world is covered in a serene white blanket, Rob and I know there's a good chance we might be snowed in. On these days, we embrace the slower pace of life, even if it only lasts a little while.

Bundled up in their winter coats, the kids cannot wait to be the first ones to make footprints on the blank white canvas. As they build snowmen in the yard, chase each other around with snowballs, and make snow angels, I know it's only a matter of time before they come back inside requesting a mug of rich hot chocolate.

There's something about snow days that always inspires me to make perfectly grilled cheese sandwiches to go along with a bowl of hot, creamy tomato soup. The simplicity of the meal captures the essence of our day so well.

By bedtime I stare out the window one last time, taking in the beautiful contrast between the light snowflakes and the dark night sky. I close my eyes, thankful for the peace I feel in the calmness of my surroundings, and remember why I love snow days so much.

# Hearty Beef Stew

Nothing comforts more than hearty beef stew on a blistery cold day. I love breaking apart pieces of warm rustic bread and dipping them in the rich, flavorful broth. With every bite I feel nourished. The best part: it tastes even better the next day!

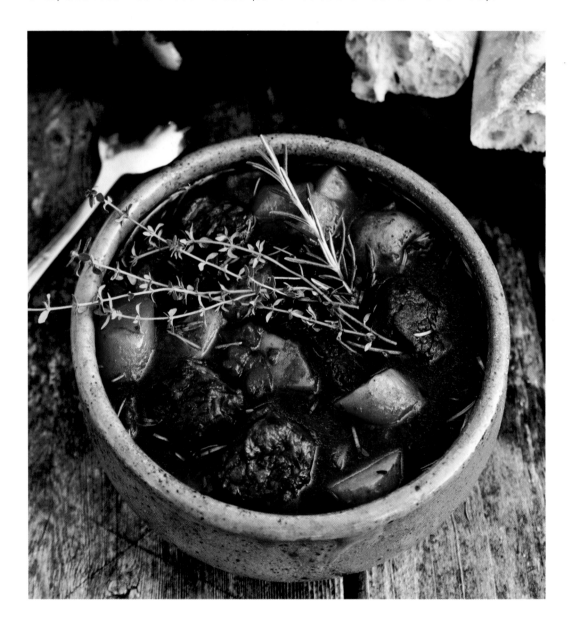

1. Combine the flour, salt, and pepper in a large bowl. Toss the beef in the flour mixture until completely coated.

2. In a large Dutch oven or soup pot, heat the oil over medium-high heat. Add a third of the beef pieces and cook until browned on all sides, a total of 8 to 10 minutes, making sure not to overcrowd the beef in the pot. Transfer the cooked beef to a medium bowl. Adding more oil if necessary, brown the remaining meat in 2 additional batches, moving each cooked batch to the medium bowl.

3. Heat 1 tablespoon of oil in the pot, and add the onions, garlic, and celery. Sauté for 2 minutes. (Don't worry if a dark brown, crusted residue has formed on the bottom of the pot.) Add the wine, balsamic vinegar, and sugar, and stir with a wooden spoon, scraping the bottom of the pot until all the residue has dissolved.

4. Stir in the beef broth, chicken bouillon cubes, tomatoes with the liquid, potatoes, carrots, rosemary, and thyme. Return the cooked beef to the pot. Bring the stew to a boil and then reduce the heat to a simmer. Cover the pot and cook until the beef is tender, about 1½ hours.

*Got a slow-cooker?* After coating the stew beef in flour, add the beef and all the other ingredients to a large slow-cooker. Cook for 7 to 10 hours on low heat or for 4 hours on high heat.

SERVES 6 TO 8

⅓ cup all-purpose flour

1 tablespoon kosher salt

1 tablespoon freshly ground black pepper

3 pounds beef stew meat

3 tablespoons vegetable oil or olive oil, plus more if needed

1 medium onion, coarsely chopped

4 garlic cloves, chopped

3 celery ribs, sliced crosswise into ½-inch pieces

½ cup red wine

¼ cup balsamic vinegar

¼ cup granulated sugar

Two 14-ounce cans beef broth

3 chicken-flavored bouillon cubes

One 14-ounce can diced tomatoes

1 pound small red potatoes, quartered

3 carrots, peeled and sliced crosswise into 1-inch pieces

1 teaspoon dried rosemary

1 teaspoon dried thyme

# Spiced Pumpkin Butter

Late fall would not be complete without making several batches of yummy spiced pumpkin butter. The autumn aroma wafting through the house is an added pleasure from this homemade pumpkin treat. I love spreading spoonfuls of it on my morning toast, but my favorite way to eat pumpkin butter is as a dessert topping over vanilla ice cream with a sprinkling of granola. Oh my goodness—it's amazing!

**MAKES 4 CUPS**

**One 29-ounce can pure pumpkin puree**

**1½ cups apple juice**

**1 cup granulated sugar**

**¾ cup firmly packed dark brown sugar**

**1 tablespoon pumpkin pie spice**

Combine all the ingredients in a large heavy pot, and bring to a boil over medium-high heat. Reduce the heat to very low and simmer for 1 hour, stirring the mixture every 20 minutes to keep it from burning. Serve warm or cold. Store in a sealed jar for up to 2 weeks.

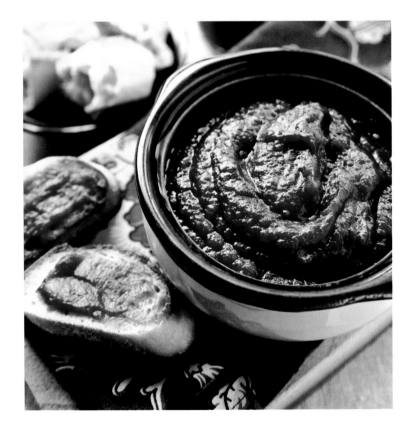

# Creamy Tomato Soup

Through years of eating canned tomato soup, it never occurred to me that I could make it at home—until I did. I was amazed to see how easy it was to prepare and how truly delicious it tasted—especially compared to the canned version. I love to make this soup throughout the year, enjoying it with a warm grilled cheese sandwich or all by itself.

1. In a large heavy pot, heat the olive oil over medium heat. Add the onions, sugar, and salt. Cook for 10 minutes, or until the onions are translucent and soft. Stir in the diced tomatoes with the liquid and the chicken broth. Bring the soup to a boil; then turn the heat to low and simmer gently for 15 minutes.

2. Pour in the cream, and using an immersion blender, puree the soup until smooth. (If you do not have an immersion blender, carefully pour the soup into a blender, filling it no more than three-quarters full and venting the lid to allow the steam to escape. Be careful not to fill the blender to the top or tomato soup will explode all over your kitchen! Puree until smooth. Return the soup to the pot and reheat if necessary.)

*My favorite tomatoes:* San Marzano tomatoes are noticeably sweeter and richer in flavor than other varieties. Although they may be slightly more expensive than the more common types, the incredible fresh flavor is worth the extra money.

**SERVES 6**

1 tablespoon olive oil

1 medium onion, chopped

1 tablespoon granulated sugar

¼ teaspoon kosher salt

One 29-ounce can diced tomatoes (I love San Marzano tomatoes)

One 14-ounce can chicken broth

½ cup heavy cream

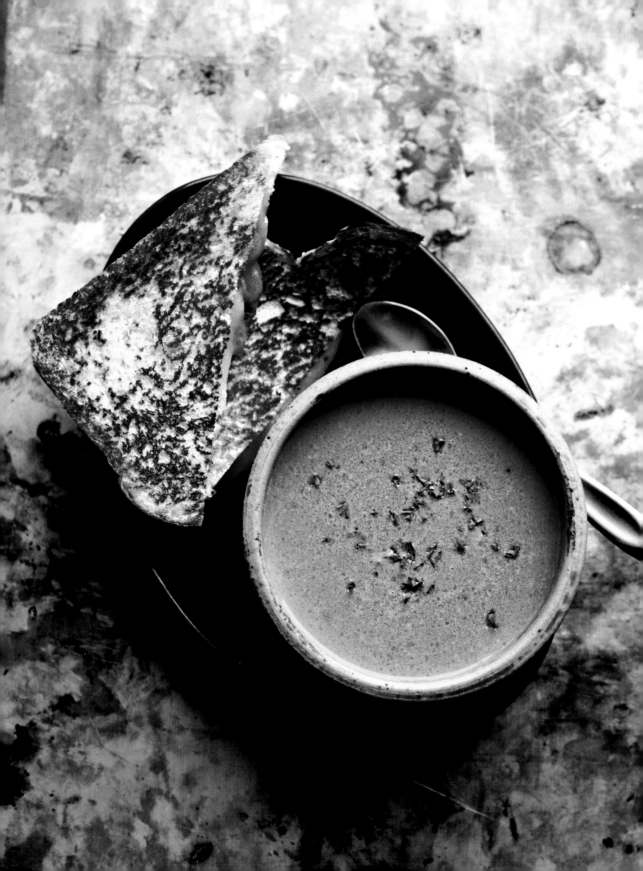

# Grilled Cheese Sandwiches

Is there anything tastier than warm melted cheddar cheese oozing out between slices of buttery toasted bread? I don't think so. I never get tired of eating grilled cheese sandwiches, especially when they're dipped in creamy tomato soup. Every time I eat one, I'm reminded why I love it so much!

Heat a nonstick or cast-iron skillet (I don't recommend using stainless steel for this recipe) over medium-low heat. Spread ½ tablespoon of the butter on one side of each slice of bread. Lay 1 slice of bread in the skillet, buttered side down. Spread ½ cup of the shredded cheese over the bread. Place another slice of bread on top, buttered side up. Cook each side of the sandwich until it is golden brown and the cheese is beginning to melt. Repeat to make the other 3 sandwiches. Cut each sandwich into halves and serve.

*Just for fun:* Instead of cutting the sandwiches in half, cut them into 1-inch squares and serve them as grilled cheese croutons on top of bowls of tomato soup.

*Variations:* If you're feeling more adventurous, substitute smoked Gouda for the cheddar cheese, or try thinly sliced sourdough or rustic bread.

**SERVES 4**

**4 tablespoons (½ stick) unsalted butter, at room temperature**

**8 slices white bread**

**2 cups (one 8-ounce package) shredded cheddar cheese**

# Rich Hot Chocolate

If you've never made homemade hot chocolate, you're missing out on one of life's greatest pleasures. The indulgence of rich chocolate infused with cream will make you feel special and pampered from the very first sip!

**SERVES 6**

**One 12-ounce bag semisweet chocolate chips**

**5 cups milk**

**1 cup heavy cream**

**½ teaspoon kosher salt**

In a medium saucepan, combine the chocolate chips, milk, cream, and salt. Heat over medium heat until the liquid begins to form tiny bubbles. Reduce the heat to a low simmer. Whisk the mixture until the chocolate has completed melted and is thoroughly blended in. Serve immediately.

*Note of caution:* Make sure the milk doesn't boil over. As milk heats up, it starts to foam and quickly bubbles over—a surefire way to make a mess on the stove.

*Just for fun:* Top off each mug of hot chocolate with whipped cream and a pinch of ground cinnamon or chocolate shavings.

*Variation:* Add a shot of espresso for the best mocha you'll ever taste.

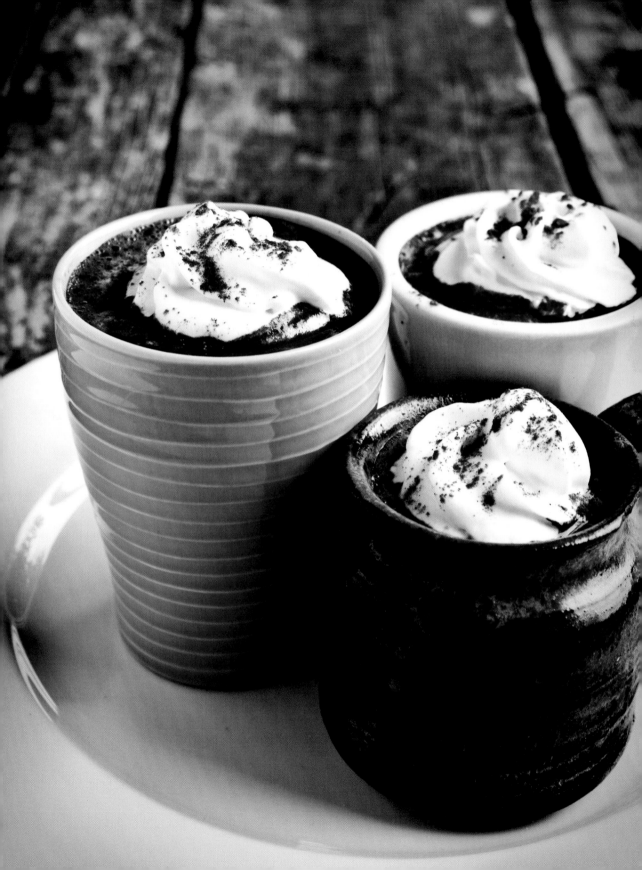

# Soft Chocolate Gingersnap Cookies

Wrap yourself in a cozy blanket and curl up near the fire with a batch of these cookies. They're a comforting treat and the perfect pick-me-up when the weather is gloomy. I like eating them right out of the oven while they're still warm. Pair the cookies with a cup of hot orange spice black tea for an extra-special treat.

**MAKES 24 MEDIUM COOKIES**

2 cups all-purpose flour

3 tablespoons unsweetened cocoa powder

¼ teaspoon salt

½ teaspoon baking soda

1 teaspoon ground cinnamon

1 teaspoon ground ginger

½ teaspoon ground cloves

½ teaspoon cream of tartar

¼ teaspoon ground nutmeg

8 tablespoons (1 stick) unsalted butter, at room temperature

¾ cup firmly packed dark brown sugar

½ cup plus ⅓ cup granulated sugar

1 egg

¼ cup molasses

1. Preheat the oven to 350°F. Line a baking sheet with parchment paper.

2. In a medium bowl, whisk together the flour, cocoa powder, salt, baking soda, cinnamon, ginger, cloves, cream of tartar, and nutmeg. Set aside.

3. In a mixing bowl, cream the butter, brown sugar, and the ½ cup granulated sugar on medium-high speed for 2 minutes, or until fluffy. Reduce the speed to medium and beat in the egg and molasses for 30 seconds. Scrape down the sides and bottom of the bowl and beat for an additional 30 seconds. Slowly add the dry ingredients to the wet ingredients, mixing just until incorporated.

4. Using a medium cookie scoop, form 1½-inch balls of dough. Coat the balls in the remaining ⅓ cup granulated sugar, and place them about 2 inches apart on the baking sheet. Bake for 14 to 16 minutes; the cookies will be slightly rounded and cracked on top.

5. Remove the cookies from the oven and let them cool on the baking sheet for 5 minutes. Then carefully lift the parch-

ment paper from the baking sheet and transfer the cookies and parchment to a wire rack to finish cooling.

*Just for fun:* Sandwich a scoop of vanilla ice cream between 2 cookies for an unusual gingery ice cream sandwich.

*Substitution:* Turbinado (raw) sugar can be substituted for the granulated sugar.

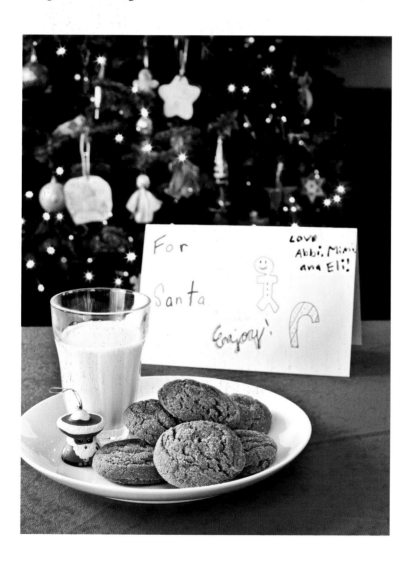

# fourteen

# CHRISTMAS MORNING

Christmas mornings in our house are quite the frenzy, and that's putting it mildly. I'm usually awakened from my grogginess by the pitter-patter of small feet running toward our bedroom with one daughter yelling at the other, "Wake up! Santa was here!" The next thing I know, I'm being tossed around like popcorn as the kids jump on our bed, fueled by pure adrenaline, anticipation, and joy. It's a game to them, and so far they're winning. As each child pleads with us to wake up, my own excitement starts to grow. I think of how enjoyable it will be to see the looks on my beloved children's faces as they open presents and hold each gift up as if it's a prized trophy.

But before the wrapping paper is torn and ribbons are undone, there are two very important things on my mind: coffee and breakfast, in that order. The smell of freshly brewed coffee is a welcome aroma for a sleepy mom of three who stayed up way too late Christmas Eve, wrapping presents and preparing sweet yeasted dough for breakfast. With the oven preheating, I grab two mugs of eggnog coffees and rejoin the rest of the family just in time to share in the joy of opening presents. Each child squeals in delight as they take turns opening gifts, and it's not long before they're joined by the sound of a beeping oven, announcing that it's ready to bake our Christmas breakfast. I break away again for just a minute to place a hearty breakfast casserole and a beautiful batch of fluffy cinnamon rolls into the oven. After

I close the door, I slip back into my chair and I take in the rest of the morning festivities.

There's something magical about sharing straight-from-the-oven cinnamon rolls with loved ones, especially on Christmas morning. The alluring aroma, inviting sight, and pillowy, melt-in-your-mouth texture imparts a memorable feeling of family togetherness. These familiar moments are the kind my kids will be coming home to years after they've moved out of the house. They are also permanently engraved on my heart, and make waking up at the crack of dawn and being tossed around like popcorn totally worth it.

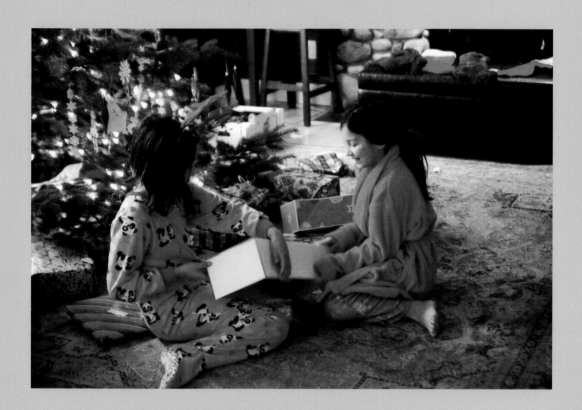

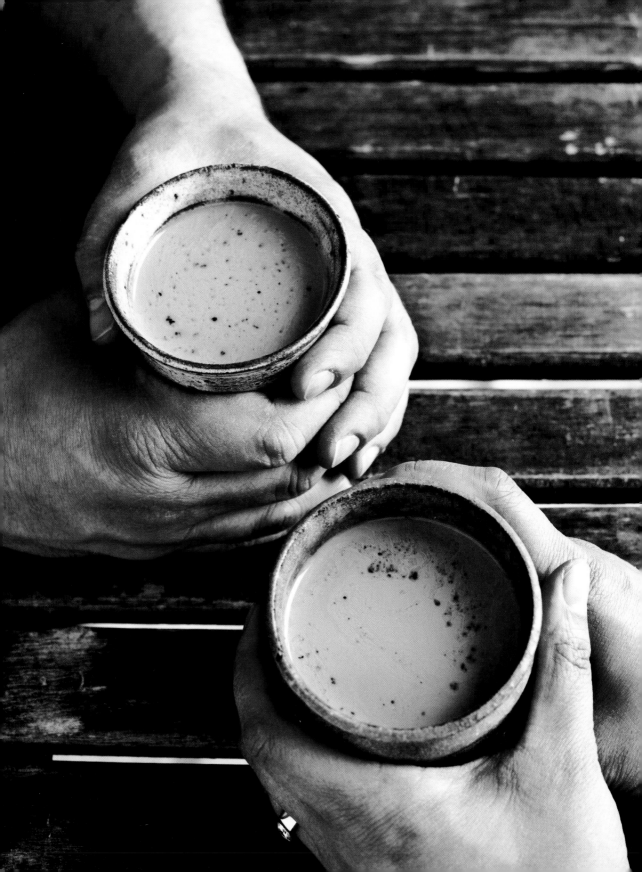

# Eggnog Coffee

During the winter I rely on eggnog coffees to put me in the holiday spirit and get me through the season. Inspired by the latte version, I discovered I could save some money and make my own at home. And guess what? I actually like mine better.

Heat the eggnog in the microwave oven for 45 seconds. Add the coffee and nutmeg. Sweeten it with a little sugar if necessary, and if you like, top it off with a dollop of whipped cream.

*Just for fun:* Turn this into a dessert beverage by adding a scoop or two of vanilla ice cream for an eggnog affogato-like treat!

**SERVES 1**

½ cup eggnog

¾ cup double-strength hot brewed coffee

Pinch of ground nutmeg

Granulated sugar, if needed

Whipped cream (optional)

# Gingerbread Pumpkin Waffles

In my twenties, one of my favorite Saturday-morning rituals was meeting friends for breakfast. We would often go to a restaurant called Jitterbug, which served the most amazing spiced gingerbread waffles. Although Jitterbug has since closed its doors, I still enjoy good gingerbread waffles—especially this pumpkin version.

**MAKES 8 WAFFLES**

1½ cups all-purpose flour

½ cup granulated sugar

1 tablespoon baking powder

1½ teaspoons ground cinnamon

1 teaspoon ground ginger

½ teaspoon ground cloves

¼ teaspoon salt

1 cup whole milk

½ cup pure pumpkin puree

¼ cup molasses

4 tablespoons (½ stick) unsalted butter, at room temperature

¼ cup vegetable oil

1. Heat a waffle maker to high heat.

2. In a large bowl, whisk together the flour, sugar, baking powder, cinnamon, ginger, cloves, and salt. Add the milk, pumpkin, molasses, butter, and oil, and stir until the batter is smooth.

3. Spray the waffle maker with nonstick cooking spray, and spoon ½ cup of the batter into each mold. Close the cover and cook for 8 to 10 minutes for crisp waffles. Repeat with the rest of the batter. (You can keep the cooked waffles on a baking sheet in a low oven while you prepare the rest of them.)

*Cook's note:* My waffle maker has an automatic timer to let me know when the waffles are ready. Because these waffles are slightly denser than regular waffles, the cooking time is longer than the automated alert. Your cooking time may vary, depending on your waffle maker. If you like a crisp shell, as I do, continue to cook the waffles until no more steam puffs from the waffle maker.

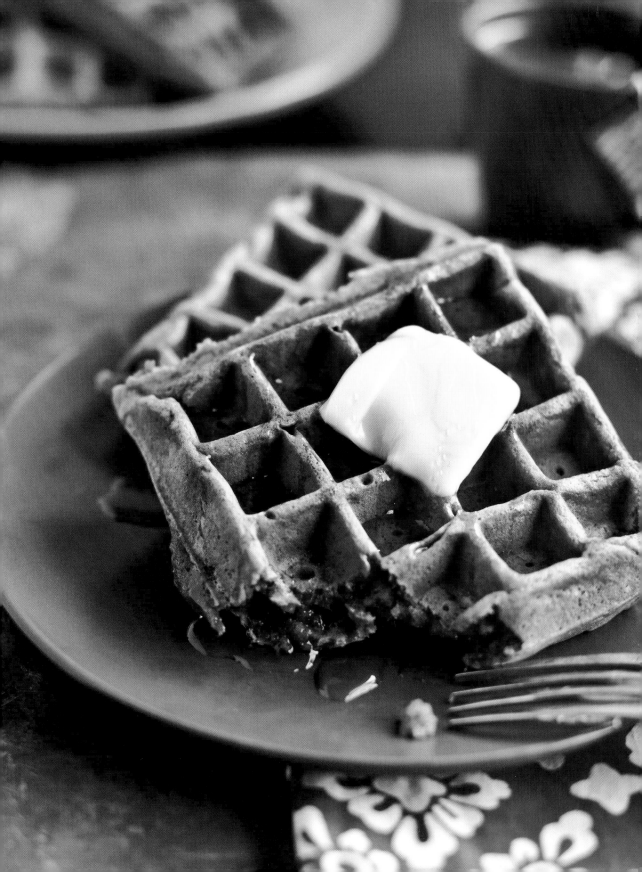

# Stuffed Apple Pie French Toast

Inspired by my very first contributing post for The Pioneer Woman's TastyKitchen.com site, I came up with my own variation on this fun breakfast dish, combining two of my favorite foods: apple pie à la mode and French toast. The spiced apple–infused maple syrup is amazing, and I'm convinced you could even serve this dish for dessert!

**SERVES 12**

4 tablespoons (½ stick) unsalted butter

2 tablespoons granulated sugar

1 tablespoon plus 1 teaspoon ground cinnamon

⅛ teaspoon ground nutmeg

2 Granny Smith apples, peeled, cored, and cut into ½-inch cubes

8 ounces (1 cup) cream cheese, at room temperature

½ cup pure maple syrup

½ cup milk

2 eggs

1 teaspoon pure vanilla extract

1 loaf French bread, cut into twelve 2-inch-thick slices

Confectioners' sugar

Candied Pecans (page 217), coarsely chopped

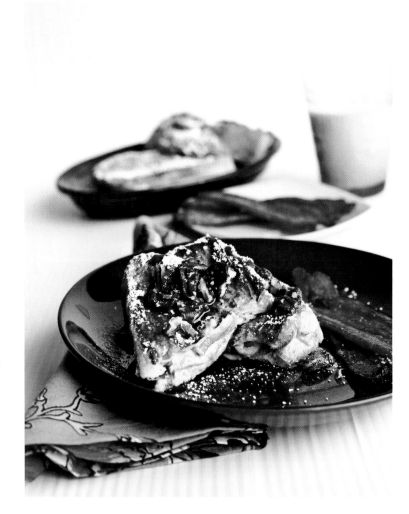

1. In a small pot, melt the butter over medium heat. Add ¼ cup water, the sugar, the 1 teaspoon cinnamon, and the nutmeg, and stir until well mixed. Add the apples and toss until they are coated in the syrup. Cook the mixture for 5 minutes, or until the apples are slightly soft but still firm. Strain the apple mixture over a bowl, and reserve the liquid. In another bowl, mix the cooked apples thoroughly with the cream cheese, and set aside. Combine the reserved liquid with the maple syrup, and transfer it to a syrup dispenser or small serving pitcher.

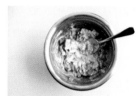

2. In an 8 x 8-inch shallow baking dish, whisk the milk, eggs, vanilla, and remaining 1 tablespoon cinnamon until well combined.

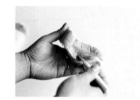

3. Cutting from the bottom of each piece of bread, create a 2- to 3-inch pocket for the filling. Spoon 3 to 4 tablespoons of the apple–cream cheese mixture into each pocket. Set the stuffed bread on a baking sheet.

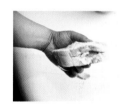

4. Heat a nonstick frying pan or griddle over medium heat, and grease it with nonstick cooking spray. Working in batches, dip both sides of each stuffed bread slice in the egg mixture, being careful not to dip more bread than will fit in the frying pan at one time. Cook the bread on each side for 3 to 5 minutes, or until golden brown. Repeat with the rest of the stuffed bread.

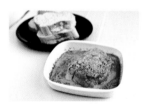

5. Serve the French toast with a light dusting of confectioners' sugar, a sprinkling of candied pecans, and a drizzle of the apple cinnamon–infused syrup. Any leftover apple cream cheese can be served on the side.

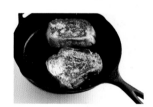

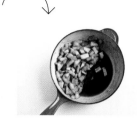

*Cook's note:* I like to keep my French toast slices warm by placing them on a plate and wrapping it in aluminum foil. Every time I finish cooking a batch, I add the slices to the warm plate, remembering to cover it back up with foil.

*Just for fun:* Serve this breakfast for dessert by topping each slice with a scoop of vanilla ice cream.

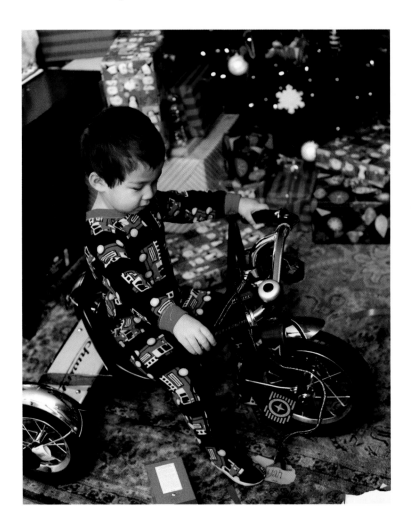

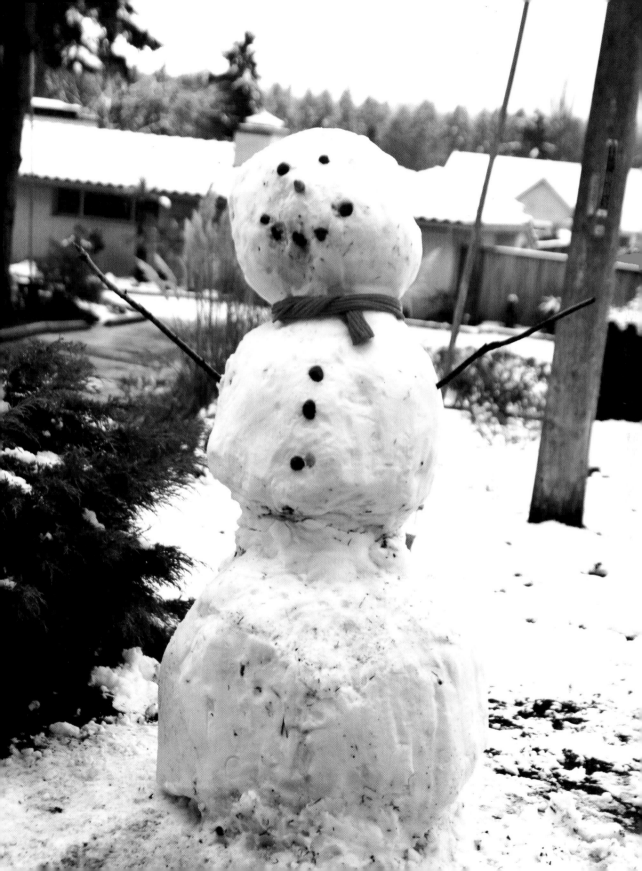

# Cinnamon Rolls

Who can resist the lure of homemade cinnamon rolls straight from the oven? Baking these sweet, pillowy rolls is a Christmas tradition that my kids look forward to every year.

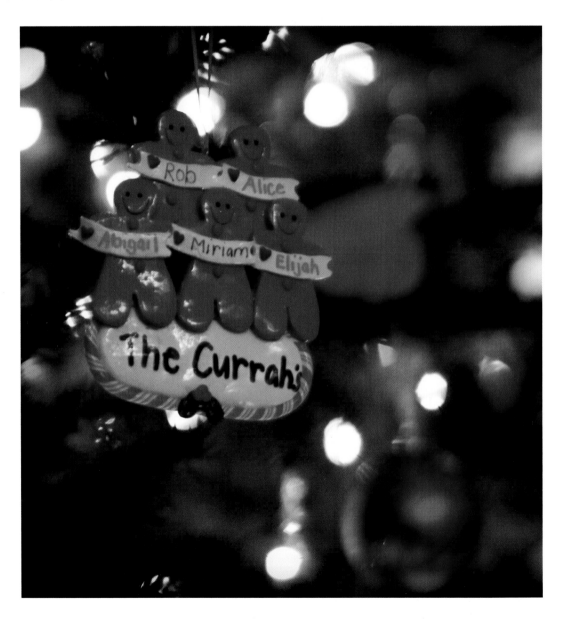

1. To make the dough, combine the milk, egg, melted butter, oil, sugar, and salt in the bowl of a stand mixer fitted with the dough hook. Cover the liquid mixture with the flour, and then sprinkle the yeast on the very top. Knead the mixture on low to medium speed until the dough is smooth and elastic, 5 to 7 minutes, adding more flour as needed so that the dough does not stick to the bowl and does not look wet. Place the dough in a large buttered bowl and cover it with a damp towel. Allow the dough to rise in a warm area until it has doubled in size, about 1 hour.

2. Butter a 9 x 10-inch baking pan. To make the filling, combine the granulated sugar, brown sugar, and cinnamon in a small bowl, and set aside.

3. When the dough has risen, turn it onto a lightly floured surface and roll it out to form a rectangle slightly larger than the baking pan. Spread the entire surface of the dough with the melted butter, and then sprinkle the cinnamon/sugar mixture on top. Use your hands to make sure the entire surface is evenly coated.

4. Starting from the long edge farthest from you, use both hands to tightly roll the dough toward you, forming a log. Pinch the end seam into the log to seal it. Cut the log into 12 equal slices and place them, flat side down, in the baking pan. Cover the pan tightly with plastic wrap and refrigerate overnight. When it's time to bake the rolls, take them out of the refrigerator and allow them to rest on the countertop for 30 minutes.

5. Meanwhile, preheat the oven to 375°F.

6. Remove the plastic wrap, and bake the rolls for 20 minutes, or until golden brown.

SERVES 12

DOUGH

1 cup warm milk (115°F)

1 egg, slightly beaten, at room temperature

4 tablespoons (½ stick) unsalted butter, melted

¼ cup vegetable oil

½ cup granulated sugar

½ teaspoon salt

3½ cups all-purpose flour, plus more for dusting

One packet (2¼ teaspoons) instant dry yeast

FILLING

½ cup granulated sugar

½ cup firmly packed dark brown sugar

3 tablespoons ground cinnamon

8 tablespoons (1 stick) unsalted butter, melted

ICING

1 cup confectioners' sugar, sifted

4 tablespoons (½ stick) unsalted butter, at room temperature

¼ cup cream cheese, at room temperature

1 teaspoon pure vanilla extract

¼ teaspoon salt

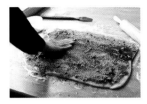

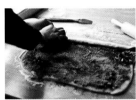

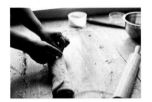

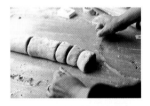

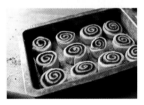

**7.** While the rolls are baking, make the icing: Using a hand or stand mixer, mix the confectioners' sugar, butter, cream cheese, vanilla, and salt on low speed until the sugar is fully absorbed. Increase the speed to medium and whip the icing for 2 minutes.

**8.** Spread the frosting over the cinnamon rolls while they are still warm. Serve immediately.

*Helping the dough to rise:* While the dough is being kneaded in the stand mixer, I preheat my oven to 200°F. I turn the oven off when the dough is ready, and then I place my covered bowl in the oven and leave the oven door cracked open. This helps the dough rise more quickly.

*Cutting the roll into pieces:* I use dental floss to cut raw cinnamon roll dough cleanly into individual rolls. Using a 12-inch-long piece of unflavored floss, center the floss underneath the log of cinnamon roll dough with the ends pointing away from the dough. Grab each end of the floss and cross one end over the other. Quickly pull the ends away from the log to cut a clean slice.

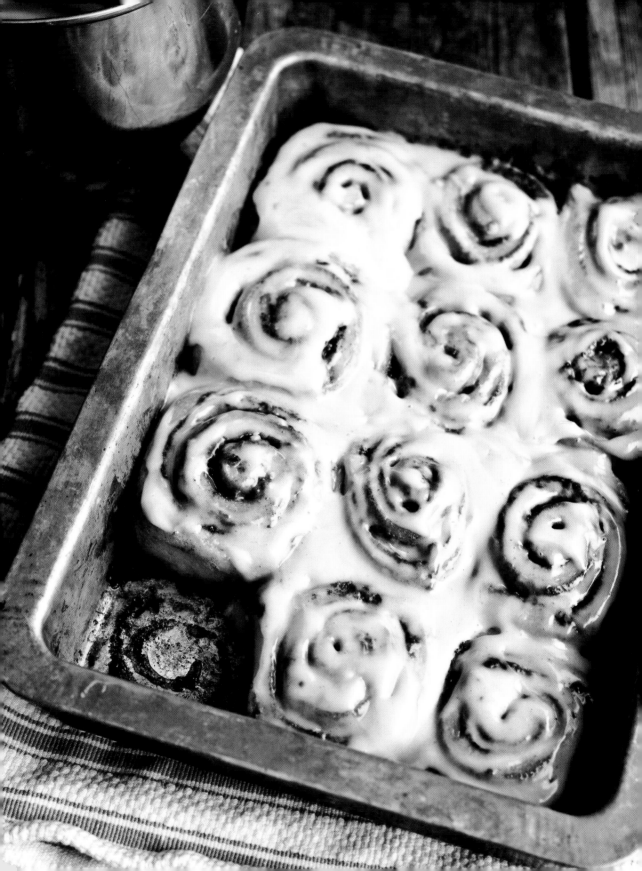

# Christmas Breakfast Casserole

I love this breakfast casserole for so many reasons: savory crumbled sausage, mushrooms, potatoes, and eggs to name a few. But what I love most is the fact that I can prepare it the night before and then just pop it in the oven in the morning. This dish could easily be called "The Disappearing Casserole" because there usually are only crumbs left when I serve it to friends and family.

**SERVES 6 TO 8**

1 pound sweet Italian sausage meat, crumbled

½ onion, chopped

One 8-ounce package sliced mushrooms

2 cups frozen Tater Tots (unthawed)

6 slices white bread, cut into large pieces

3 cups grated extra-sharp cheddar cheese

8 eggs

1 cup heavy cream

1½ cups whole milk

1 teaspoon Dijon mustard

½ teaspoon kosher salt

½ teaspoon freshly ground black pepper

1 tomato, thinly sliced

3 tablespoons chopped fresh parsley

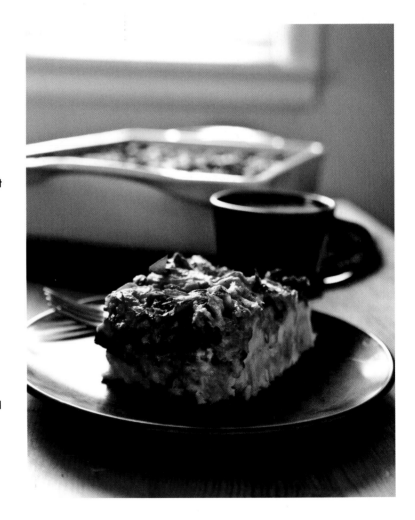

1. In a medium skillet over medium heat, brown the sausage, onions, and mushrooms together until the sausage is no longer pink. Set aside.

2. Spray a 9 x 13-inch casserole dish with nonstick cooking spray. Cover the bottom of the casserole dish with the Tater Tots, followed by the bread. Spread the sausage mixture evenly over the bread, and top with the cheese.

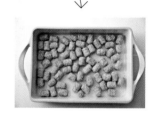

3. In a medium bowl, whisk together the eggs, cream, milk, mustard, salt, and pepper. Pour the egg mixture over the ingredients in the casserole. Layer the top of the casserole with the tomatoes, and sprinkle with the parsley. Cover it with plastic wrap and refrigerate overnight.

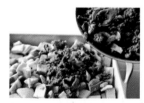

4. The next morning, remove the casserole from the refrigerator and preheat the oven to 350°F.

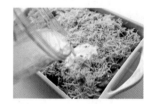

5. When the oven is ready, remove the plastic wrap and bake the casserole, uncovered, for 1 hour, or until it is bubbly and browned around the edges.

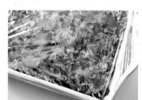

*Variations:* Feel free to substitute cooked bacon, ham, or seasoned ground beef for the sausage, or to use no meat at all for a vegetarian version. Other add-ins include chopped bell peppers, black olives, sliced zucchini, and/or spinach.

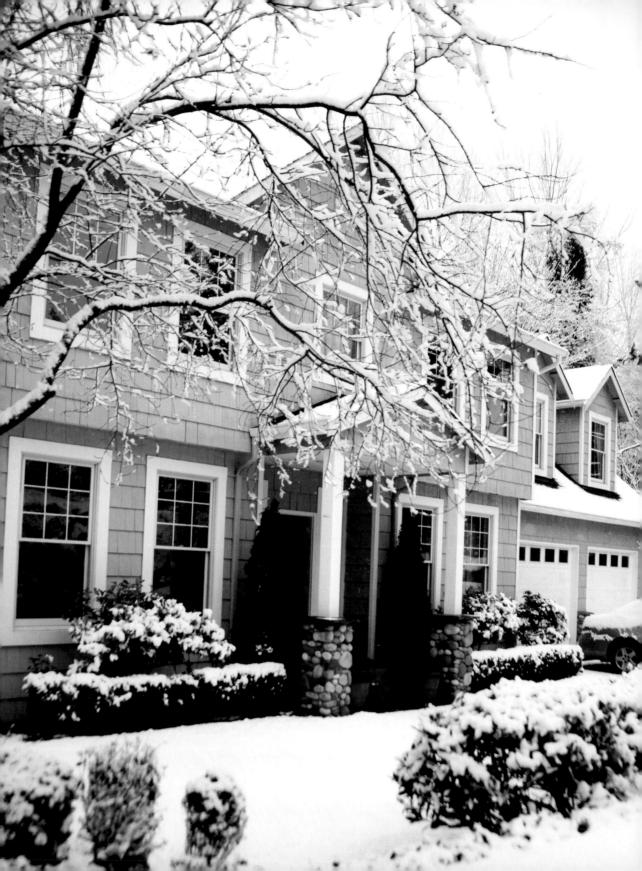

# fifteen

# HOLIDAY GET-TOGETHER

Walk by our house the day after Thanksgiving and you'll find Rob with his arms stretched to the rooftop in a web of Christmas lights. The annual hanging of the lights signals the beginning of the holiday season for my family, and when darkness falls and I go outside to look, the sight of our home all lit up always fills me with awe. Bright lights serve as magical eye candy, and I love how they make our home look as whimsical and festive as a gingerbread house.

With spice-scented candles lit, a fire burning in our woodstove, and Vince Guaraldi's *A Charlie Brown Christmas* playing in the background, a cozy warmth permeates the air. These small touches help us to embrace the holidays with open arms and celebratory hearts.

I love preparing and serving food to enhance the ambience of the season. Eating, laughing, and enjoying holiday cheer in the presence of friends and family—that's what I look forward to each year.

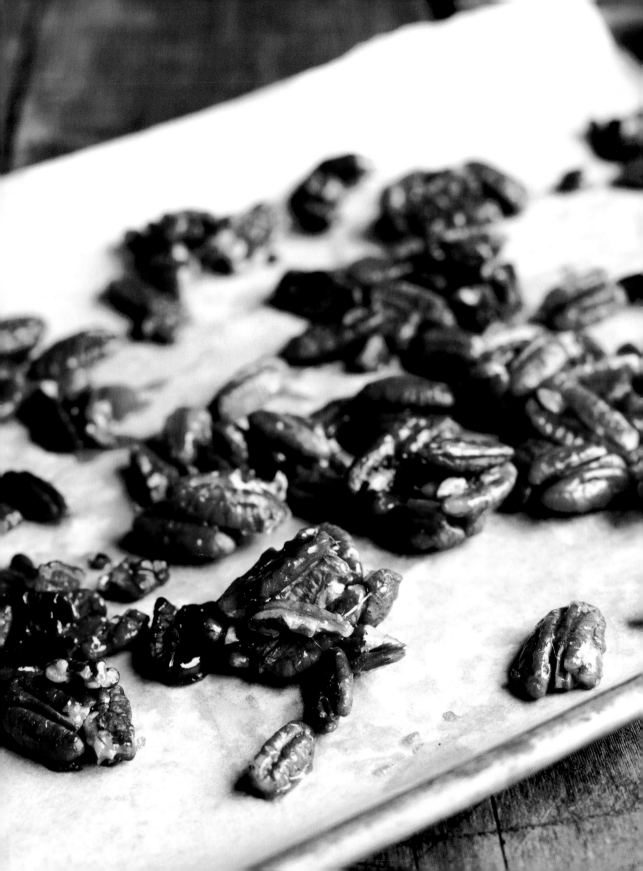

# Candied Pecans

I love adding candied pecans to baked goods, salads, and other sweet or savory dishes—they add a special touch to just about anything. When I'm not eating them straight out of the bowl, I like to give them away as hostess gifts. I use these pecans in my recipes for Pear Gorgonzola Pecan Salad (page 174) and Overnight Baked French Toast Casserole (page 24).

1. Line a baking sheet with parchment paper.

2. Heat the sugar and 2 tablespoons of water in a small nonstick saucepan over medium-high heat, stirring with a wooden spoon until the sugar has dissolved. Watch attentively while the sugar syrup gently bubbles and changes from clear to a honey color. Once the syrup has changed color, add the pecans and salt. Stir for 1 minute, until the nuts are coated with syrup.

3. Immediately spread the pecans out in a single layer on the baking sheet. Separate the pecans as best you can with 2 forks, but don't worry if a few of them are clustered. Allow the pecans to cool completely before storing them in an airtight container. They will keep for up to 2 weeks.

*Variations:* Add ¼ teaspoon cayenne pepper along with the pecans for a spicier kick.

**MAKES 1 CUP**

¼ cup granulated sugar

1 cup pecan halves

¼ teaspoon kosher salt

# Red Pepper Relish

My husband and I can easily eat this relish by the spoonful. I particularly love pairing it with cream cheese, but you could also use a fancier cheese such as a baked Brie or Camembert. Serve the cheese and relish with your favorite crackers, and you have a great appetizer. I'm warning you in advance: this relish is very addictive!

**MAKES 1 CUP**

**1 large red bell pepper, seeded and chopped**

**½ medium onion, finely chopped**

**⅔ cup granulated sugar**

**½ cup distilled white vinegar**

**½ teaspoon red pepper flakes**

Place all the ingredients in a nonstick saucepan and cook over medium-high heat for 5 minutes, stirring occasionally. Reduce the heat to medium-low and cook for 10 minutes more, or until most of the liquid has reduced. Remove the relish from the heat and allow it to cool before serving. The relish should be kept in the refrigerator and will last for up to 2 weeks.

*Hostess gifts:* Consider making several batches and canning them in 8-ounce Mason jars to give away as hostess gifts. Homemade edible gifts are always appreciated and enjoyed!

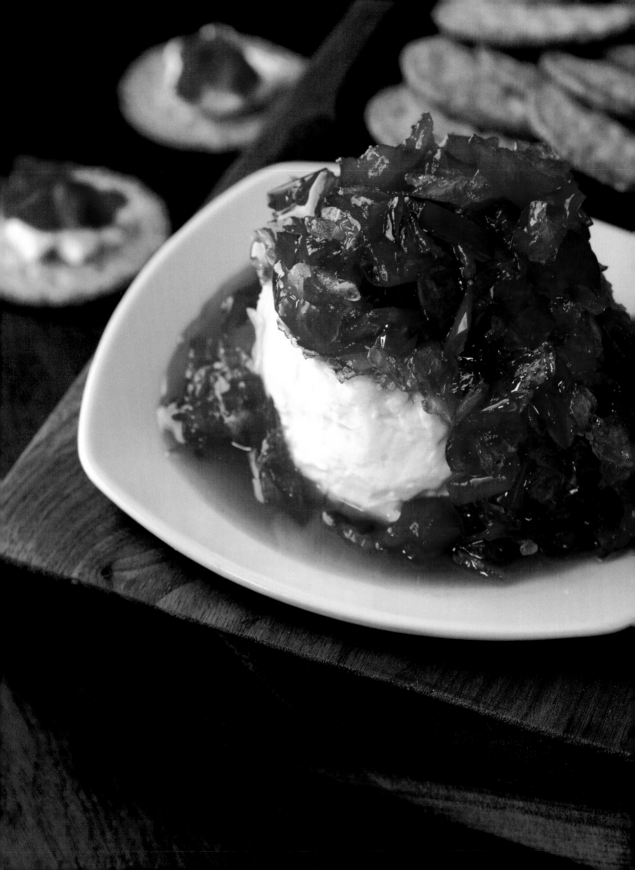

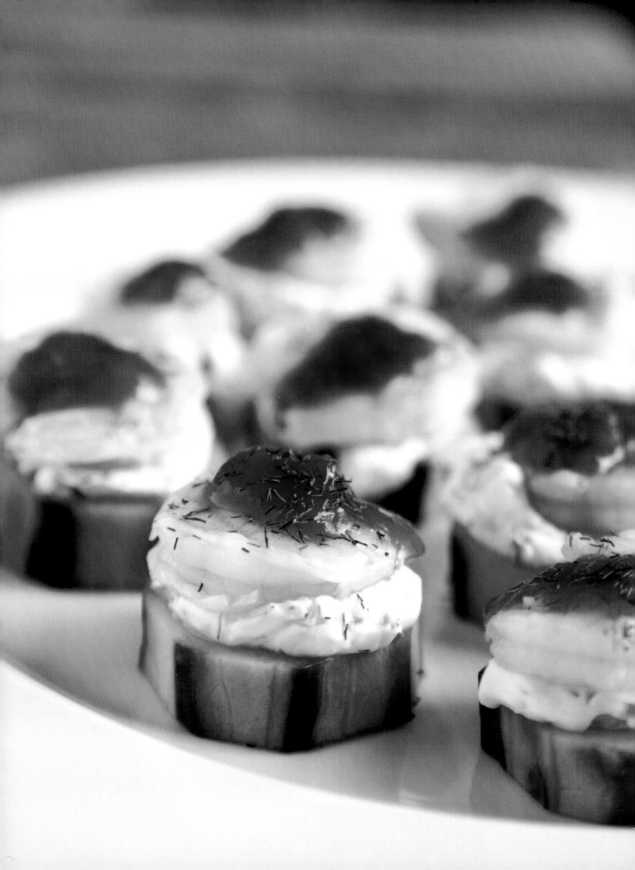

# Shrimp Cocktail Cucumber Bites

Here's my modern twist on the classic shrimp cocktail, served on top of thick cucumber slices. You'll receive accolades for making this throwback appetizer cool again!

Pat the cucumber slices dry with a paper towel. Mix the cream cheese and dill together in a small bowl. Spread 1 teaspoon of the cream cheese mixture on top of each cucumber slice. Place 1 shrimp on top of the cream cheese, and gently push it down so it adheres to the cream cheese. Place ¼ teaspoon of the cocktail sauce on top of each shrimp. Just before serving, sprinkle a pinch of dill over each shrimp cocktail bite.

*Just for fun:* Slightly hollow out each cucumber slice with a spoon to create a shallow cup. Instead of using big shrimp, mix baby shrimp with the cocktail sauce. Spread a little bit of dill cream cheese inside each cup, and then spoon the cocktail sauce on top. Top with a pinch of dill.

**MAKES 18 BITES**

1 English cucumber, peeled and cut into ⅓-inch-thick slices

4 ounces (½ cup) cream cheese, at room temperature

1 tablespoon dried dill, plus more for garnish

18 medium cocktail shrimp, cooked and shelled, tails removed

¼ cup cocktail sauce

# Teriyaki Bacon-Wrapped Pineapple Shrimp

These shrimp bites are savory, sweet, tangy, and oh so good! (As you can guess, savory and sweet is my favorite combination.) Sometimes I even serve them for dinner with a side of steamed rice.

**SERVES 8**

***Special equipment:***
**24 toothpicks**

**12 bacon slices, cut in half crosswise**

**One 14-ounce can pineapple chunks, drained**

**24 shrimp (21–25 count), shelled and deveined**

**½ cup Teriyaki Sauce (recipe follows)**

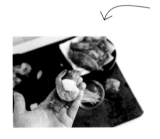

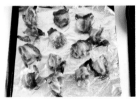

1. In a large skillet over low heat, cook the bacon until it is partially cooked but not crisp, about 5 minutes. Set the bacon aside to cool on a plate lined with paper towels.

2. Turn the broiler on high heat. Line a baking sheet with parchment paper.

3. Place a pineapple chunk in the natural curve of each shrimp. Wrap a piece of bacon around the shrimp and pineapple, and skewer with a toothpick. Place the bacon-wrapped shrimp in a single layer on the baking sheet, and broil for 4 minutes on each side, or until the shrimp are pink and firm and the outside edges of the bacon are crispy. Remove the bacon-wrapped shrimp from the broiler and generously baste each one with the teriyaki sauce before serving.

# Teriyaki Sauce

Whisk together the sugar, soy sauce, cornstarch, and ½ cup cold water in a small saucepan. Cook the sauce over medium heat for 2 minutes, stirring occasionally, until the sugar dissolves.

*Just for fun:* Substitute your favorite barbecue sauce for the teriyaki sauce, and cook the appetizers on the grill.

**MAKES 1 CUP**

½ cup granulated sugar

¼ cup reduced-sodium soy sauce

2 teaspoons cornstarch

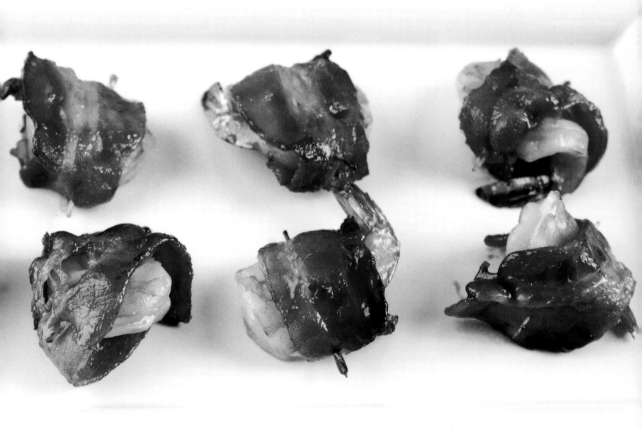

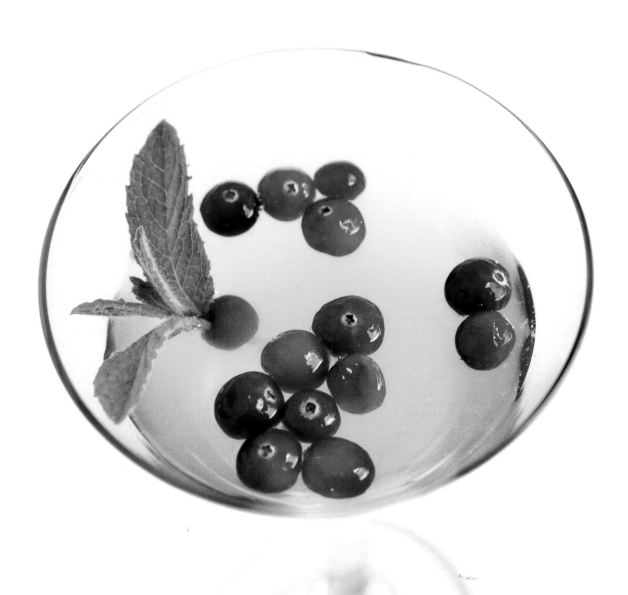

# Sparkling Cranberry Rum Punch

What better way to get into the holiday spirit than with a spiked sparkling cranberry punch? Red cranberries and green mint leaves make this festive drink cheerful and fun, with a twist of fancy. Just so you know: one glass may not seem very strong, but trust me, it packs a big punch—pun intended!

**SERVES 8**

1 cup granulated sugar

Ice cubes

6 cups seltzer water

2 cups cranberry juice cocktail

1 cup golden rum

Juice of 4 limes

1 cup fresh cranberries, plus extra for garnish

8 fresh mint sprigs, plus extra leaves for garnish

1. Bring the sugar and 1 cup water to a boil in a small saucepan. Stir until the sugar has completely dissolved. Remove the pan from the heat and allow the sugar water to cool completely.

2. Fill a large punch bowl or pitcher with 2 quarts of ice, and pour the seltzer water, cranberry juice, rum, lime juice, and sugar water over it. Give the punch a good stir, and finish it off by adding the cranberries and mint sprigs. Garnish each serving with additional cranberries and mint leaves.

*Just for fun:* Instead of fresh cranberries, use fresh pomegranate seeds as a great festive touch.

# sixteen

# CARING FOR OTHERS

For the first few days after the birth of each of my children, basic survival was my only goal. Prostrate on the sofa, I would rise only to feed the baby or take care of the other kids. Despite not showering for days (or even knowing what day it was, for that matter), I would relish the sound of the doorbell, especially at dinnertime. When a dear friend would stand in the doorway holding a warm casserole dish, that act of kindness said "You are loved" more than any greeting card ever could.

I cannot tell you how thankful our family was for the many people who brought us those meals. Their food sustained me through recovery from C-section surgery and monthlong stretches of sleep deprivation. When I look back on those first few months, they are all a blur. Thank goodness our friends and family were there to feed us. Without their help, we would have had to get along on takeout and Top Ramen.

I've been inspired to return the favor multiple times when friends have brought home a new baby or adopted a child, or when they were recovering from an illness or grieving the loss of a loved one. Words are comforting, but nothing shows you care like a hot meal delivered to the door. The thoughtfulness and kindness of others reminds me of what community is all about.

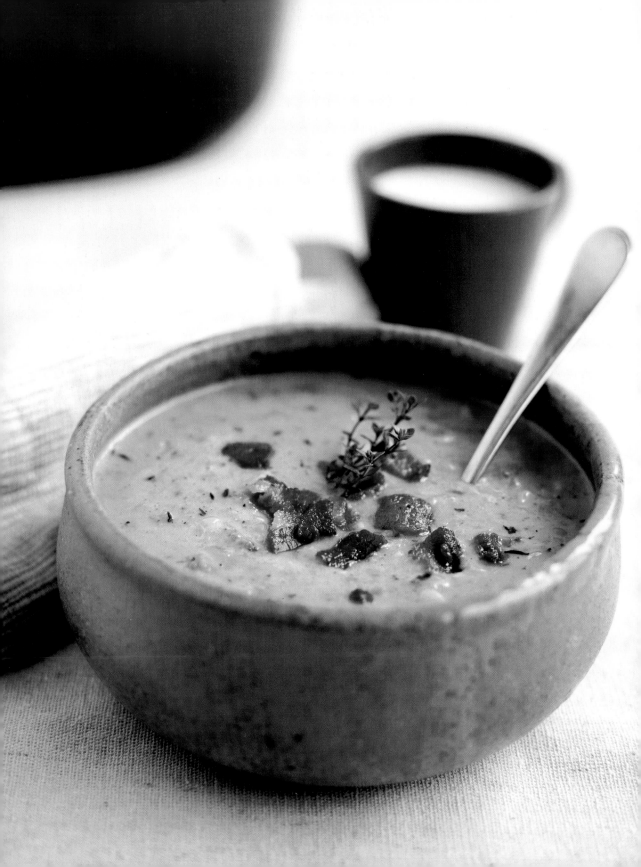

# Smoky Corn Chowder

A good corn chowder plays second fiddle to no main course—it shines on its own. And trust me: this chowder is no exception! The smokiness from the bacon and the touch of liquid smoke makes this chowder a memorable meal in need of nothing else but a spoon.

**1.** Cook the bacon in a large heavy pot over medium-high heat until it is nice and crispy. Remove the bacon with a slotted spoon and place it on a plate lined with a paper towel. Soak up all but 3 tablespoons of the bacon fat with a paper towel and discard.

**2.** Add the onions to the remaining bacon fat in the pot, and cook them over medium heat until soft, 5 to 8 minutes. Stir in the celery, red bell pepper, jalapeño pepper, garlic, crushed bouillon cubes, and thyme. Cook the vegetables for 5 minutes, stirring occasionally.

**3.** In a small bowl, whisk the heavy cream and the cornstarch together until the cornstarch is dissolved. Add the cream mixture, chicken broth, liquid smoke, potatoes, corn, and bacon to the pot. Simmer the chowder over low heat, stirring occasionally, for 20 minutes, or until the potatoes are soft and tender.

*Cook's note:* Liquid smoke is a seasoning that adds a smoky flavor to foods. It can be found in the condiment section of most grocery stores.

*Just for fun:* Adding 1 cup fresh lump crabmeat or chopped smoked salmon to the pot just before serving really elevates this to a spectacular chowder.

**SERVES 6**

½ pound thick-cut bacon, diced

1 medium onion, chopped

2 celery ribs, finely diced

1 red bell pepper, seeded and finely diced

1 jalapeño pepper, seeded and finely diced

3 garlic cloves, chopped

3 chicken bouillon cubes, crushed

1 teaspoon ground thyme

1 cup heavy cream

2 tablespoons cornstarch

4 cups chicken broth

½ teaspoon liquid smoke

4 Yukon Gold potatoes, cut into small cubes

One 16-ounce package frozen corn kernels

# Chicken Marsala

Sautéed mushrooms in a reduced Marsala sauce can transform a simple chicken dinner into a special meal without a lot of fuss. Serve this over a bed of pasta and your friends and family will insist you make it again—the ultimate compliment!

**SERVES 6**

6 skinless, boneless chicken breast halves

Kosher salt and freshly ground black pepper

½ cup all-purpose flour

¼ cup vegetable oil or extra-virgin olive oil

3 tablespoons unsalted butter

3 cups sliced fresh mushrooms

⅔ cup sweet Marsala wine

½ cup chicken broth

¼ cup dry sherry or dry white wine

¼ cup heavy cream

¼ cup chopped fresh parsley

1. Lay the chicken halves in a single layer on a cutting board. Cover the chicken with plastic wrap, and use a kitchen mallet to pound each one flat, to about ½-inch thickness. Season the chicken breasts with salt and pepper on both sides, and then dredge them in the flour.

2. Heat the oil in a large sauté pan over medium-high heat. Add the chicken breasts and cook for 4 to 5 minutes on each side, until they are golden brown. Be sure not to overcrowd the pan; work in batches if you have to. Transfer the chicken breasts to a serving platter and cover with aluminum foil. Use a paper towel to soak up any remaining oil in the sauté pan.

3. Reduce the heat under the pan to medium, and add the butter and mushrooms. Lightly season the mushrooms with salt and pepper, and sauté them for 4 to 5 minutes, until they start to brown and give off liquid. Pour in the Marsala, chicken broth, sherry, and heavy cream. Cook until the liquid has reduced by half, about 5 minutes; it will be slightly thick. Pour the mushrooms and sauce over the chicken, garnish with the parsley, and serve immediately.

*Cook's note:* Chicken Marsala can be served over your favorite pasta, rice, or sautéed vegetables.

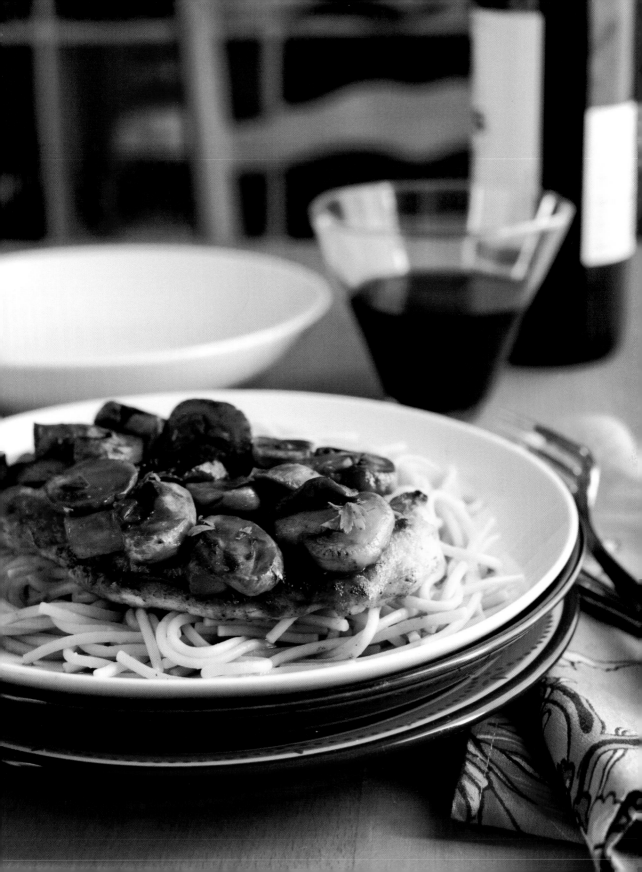

# Mulligatawny Pot Pie

It's not your grandmother's pot pie, but this creative twist on an old classic is just as comforting as the more traditional version. Inspired by the popular chicken-based curry-flavored mulligatawny soup, this dish will have you going back for seconds, and you'll love eating the leftovers (if there are any) the next day.

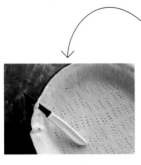

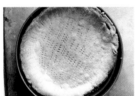

1. Preheat the oven to 450°F.

2. Spray a pie plate with nonstick cooking spray. Place one of the pie crusts in the pie plate, gently patting it against the bottom and sides, and then poke it multiple times with a fork. Carefully cut away any excess dough that is higher than the lip of the pie plate. Bake the pie crust for 20 minutes, or until it is golden brown.

3. Meanwhile, prepare the filling: Melt the butter in a heavy pot over medium heat. Add the onion and cook, stirring occasionally, until it has softened, about 5 minutes. Stir in the apple, celery, carrots, raisins, garlic, curry powder, thyme, and salt, and cook for 5 minutes, or until the vegetables have softened.

4. In a small bowl, mix the heavy cream and the cornstarch together, stirring until the cornstarch has dissolved. Raise the heat to medium-high and add the cream mixture, chicken broth, and bouillon cubes to the pot. Cook for 10 minutes, covered, stirring occasionally. Turn the heat off, and stir in the peas and chicken. The sauce should be thick enough to coat the back of the spoon; it shouldn't appear runny. If it is runny, add 2 teaspoons of additional cornstarch to 1 tablespoon cold water, mix, then add.

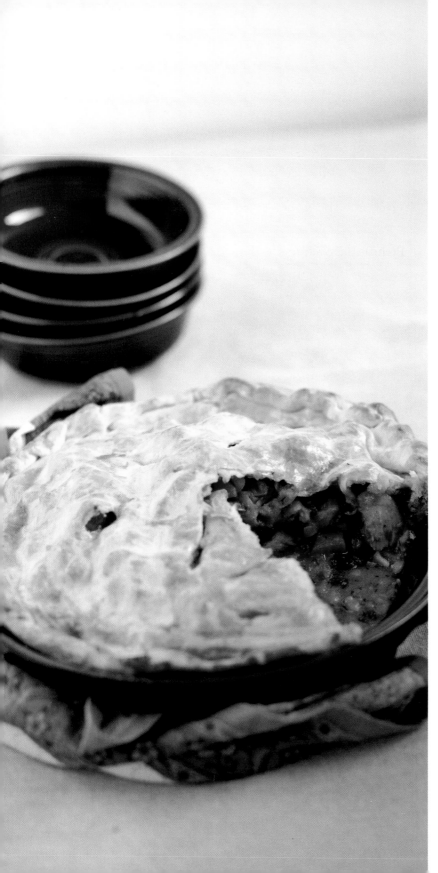

**SERVES 8**

Two 9-inch unbaked
refrigerated pie crusts

4 tablespoons (½ stick)
unsalted butter

1 medium yellow onion,
chopped

1 Granny Smith apple,
peeled, cored, and cut
into grape-size chunks

2 celery ribs, cut into
¼-inch-thick slices

2 carrots, peeled and
cut into ½-inch-thick
slices

⅓ cup raisins

3 garlic cloves,
chopped

2 tablespoons curry
powder

2 teaspoons ground
thyme

½ teaspoon kosher salt

½ cup heavy cream

3 tablespoons
cornstarch

1½ cups chicken broth

2 chicken bouillon
cubes

½ cup frozen peas

2 cups diced cooked
chicken

Egg wash: 1 egg mixed
with 1 teaspoon water
(optional)

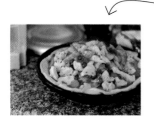

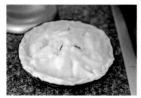

5. When the crust has finished baking, remove the pie plate from the oven. Do not worry if the baked crust is uneven around the sides. Carefully transfer the filling from the pot to the pie crust, making sure the liquid doesn't overfill the pie plate. Snugly fit the remaining unbaked crust over the filled pie, folding any excess dough over and crimping it down with your fingers just within the edge of the pie plate. Brush the crust with the egg wash, if desired. Cut 5 slits in the top crust.

6. Place the pie on a baking sheet and bake for 20 minutes, or until the top crust is golden brown. Let the pie cool for 10 minutes before serving.

*Cook's note:* I often prepare this pie using a rotisserie chicken from the deli. I'll typically double the recipe and make 2 pies—one to eat for dinner and the other to freeze for later or to give away. This way I use the whole chicken and none goes to waste.

*Double baking?* By baking the bottom crust first, you get a perfect shell to hold this pot pie together. The bottom crust will never be soggy or underbaked.

# Irresistible Ganache Brownies

I'm going to let you in on a little secret. When it comes to these brownies, allowing them to cool and set up in the refrigerator for at least 8 hours magically transforms them from really good to dangerously over-the-top good. These dense, moist, fudgy brownies are a chocolate-lover's dream.

1. Preheat the oven to 350°F. Evenly coat an 8 x 8-inch baking pan with nonstick cooking spray.

2. To make the brownies, mix the butter, granulated sugar, and brown sugar together in a medium bowl until well combined. Add the eggs and vanilla, mixing until smooth. Thoroughly mix in the cocoa powder, flour, and salt until the dry ingredients are fully incorporated. Pour the batter into the baking pan and spread it out evenly. Bake for 30 to 35 minutes, or until the center of the brownies is slightly firm to the touch and does not feel jiggly. Remove the brownies from the oven and allow them to cool completely in the pan.

3. Prepare the ganache: Pour the cream into a microwave-safe bowl and warm it the microwave for 90 seconds on full power. Remove the bowl and add the chocolate chips, stirring vigorously until the ganache is smooth and glossy. As you stir, you'll see the clumps of chocolate melt into a smooth chocolate sauce. Pour the ganache on top of the cooled brownies and spread it out with the back of a spoon. Sprinkle the chopped nuts evenly over the ganache, and gently press them down with the back of a spatula.

MAKES 16
BROWNIES

BROWNIES

12 tablespoons
(1½ sticks) unsalted
butter, melted

1¼ cups granulated
sugar

½ cup firmly packed
light brown sugar

3 eggs, beaten

2 teaspoons pure
vanilla extract

1 cup unsweetened
cocoa powder

¾ cup all-purpose flour

¼ teaspoon salt

GANACHE

½ cup heavy cream

¾ cup dark chocolate
chunks or chips (or
your favorite type of
chocolate)

½ cup chopped
pecans, toasted

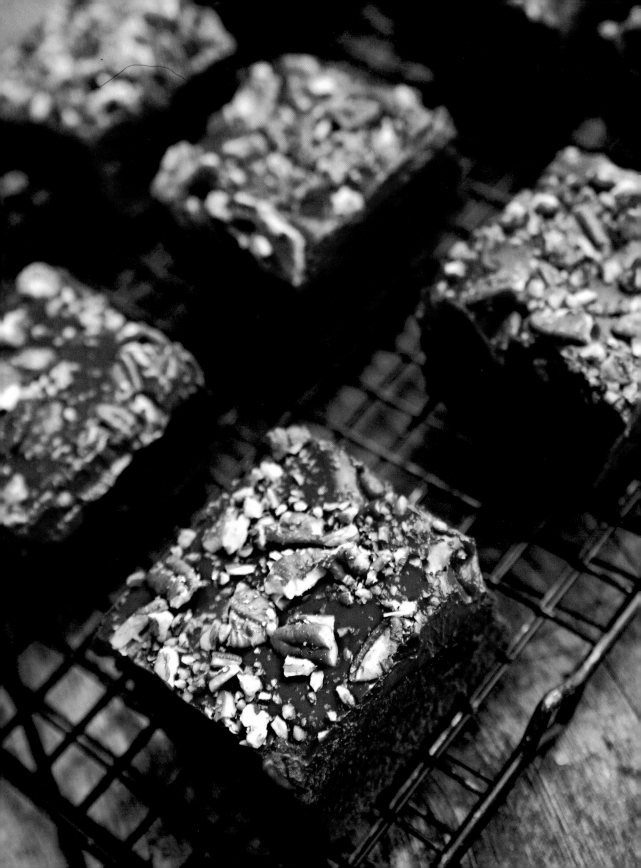

4. Allow the iced brownies to cool on the counter for 30 minutes; then cover the pan with plastic wrap, put it in the refrigerator, and leave it for at least 8 hours or overnight. Do not be tempted to cut the brownies into squares before the recommended time. This allows the texture of the brownies to change into something entirely different than if you were to cut into them right out of the oven.

5. Now that you have waited, cut the brownies into squares. You'll be rewarded with beautiful, specialty bakery–like brownies with clean cut lines. Store any uneaten brownies, covered, in the refrigerator.

*Toasting pecans:* Place the chopped pecans in a nonstick frying pan set over medium-high heat. Cook, gently shaking the pan or stirring the nuts every 30 seconds, until they are lightly toasted and fragrant, about 3 minutes.

*Cook's note:* These brownies are best served cold, straight from the refrigerator.

*Did you know?* Brownies can easily be stored in the freezer. Cut them into individual pieces and wrap each one in plastic wrap or in a snack-size zip-top plastic bag. Remove the brownies from the freezer and allow them to come to room temperature for at least 30 minutes before serving.

# seventeen

# VALENTINE'S DAY

When I was a young girl, the concept of Valentine's Day as a day for sweet-hearts always troubled me. After all, each year my classmates and I exchanged Valentine's Day cards with sayings like "Be Mine," and those silly boys were definitely *not* my sweethearts. I used to throw away the boys' cards, right after I removed the pink foil-covered chocolate heart often attached to them—who throws away free chocolate?

Twelve years of marriage and three kids later, I get it. Valentine's Day is a day to celebrate the love of family and friends, ideally over a good dinner, a bottle of wine, and a rich, chocolaty dessert to finish off the meal.

And if I'm lucky, there will be a greeting card waiting for me with the words "Be Mine" hand-written inside from my Valentine, along with a box of my favorite dark chocolate–covered caramels.

# Seared Scallops with Herbed Apricot Sauce

In my mind, scallops have always been a luxury food, reserved for special occasions. The first time I ever tried them was during a romantic sunset dinner overlooking Puget Sound. Because they can be pricey, I never trusted myself to cook them at home, convinced that I would somehow mess them up. I mean, who likes overcooked scallops? But when I finally tried cooking them at home, they were so good that I decided to prepare them as part of an annual romantic Valentine's Day dinner for my husband. Guess what? Scallops aren't hard to cook at all.

**SERVES 2 AS AN APPETIZER**

**SCALLOPS**

**6 large sea scallops, rinsed and patted dry**

**Kosher salt and freshly ground black pepper**

**1 tablespoon extra-virgin olive oil**

**1 tablespoon unsalted butter**

**HERBED APRICOT SAUCE**

**¼ cup dry white wine**

**3 tablespoons apricot preserves**

**1 garlic clove, minced**

**2 tablespoons chopped fresh flat-leaf parsley and/or chives**

**1 tablespoon unsalted butter**

**Kosher salt and freshly ground black pepper**

1. Place 2 serving plates in a warm oven.

2. Season the scallops with salt and pepper. Heat a nonstick skillet over medium-high heat and add the oil and butter. As soon as the oil-butter is hot, place the scallops in the skillet in a single layer so they are not touching each other. Sear the scallops on one side until they become opaque one-third of the way up the scallop. Then carefully turn them over and sear the other side until they become opaque one-third of the way up. The bottoms will be nicely browned. Immediately transfer the scallops to the warm serving plates.

3. To make the sauce, add the wine and apricot preserves to the skillet, whisking until well incorporated. Remove the skillet from the heat and add the garlic, parsley, and butter. Stir the sauce with a wooden spoon, and season with salt and pepper to taste. Drizzle the sauce generously over the scallops, and serve immediately.

*Cook's notes:* Make sure the scallops are as dry as possible when you add them to the skillet. This will help achieve the nice golden-brown sear you see in restaurants.

While the scallops are cooking, make sure you have all the sauce ingredients prepped and ready to go. This way the sauce can be made quickly and poured over the scallops while they are still hot.

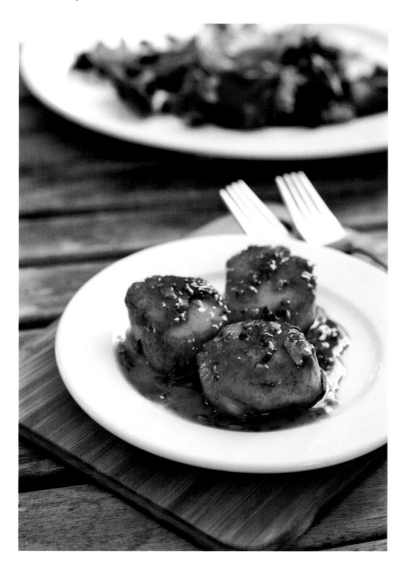

# Steamed Clams
# in White Wine

When I was young and my mother would make a big pot of steamed clams, I would wait until all the clams were eaten, then return to the pot to ladle up the rich broth. I couldn't wait to drink it straight from the bowl. Not much has changed from my mother's original recipe except that I like to add a little bit of wine—and to serve the clams with crusty bread so as not to waste a drop of that delicious broth. I especially love preparing and eating tender fresh clams after a fun day at the beach.

**SERVES 2 TO 4 AS AN APPETIZER**

3 tablespoons unsalted butter

3 garlic cloves, minced

½ cup dry white wine or dry vermouth

2 pounds littleneck or Manila clams, rinsed and scrubbed

3 tablespoons chopped fresh parsley

1 small lemon, cut into wedges

Crusty bread, for serving

Melt the butter in a large pot over medium heat. Add the garlic and cook for 1 minute, or until it is fragrant but not burned. Stir in the wine and raise the heat to medium-high. When the wine is simmering, add the clams, cover the pot, and cook, stirring occasionally, until the clams have opened, 5 to 7 minutes. Discard any closed clams. Add the parsley and give the pot a quick stir. Transfer the clams and broth to a large serving bowl, and serve the lemon wedges and bread on the side.

*Variation:* If you don't have white wine, you can substitute chicken broth.

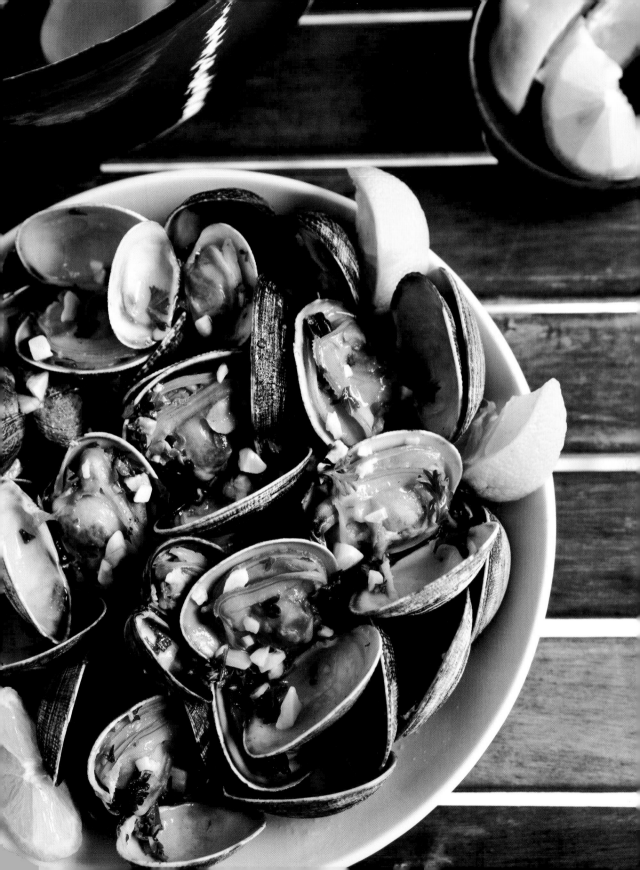

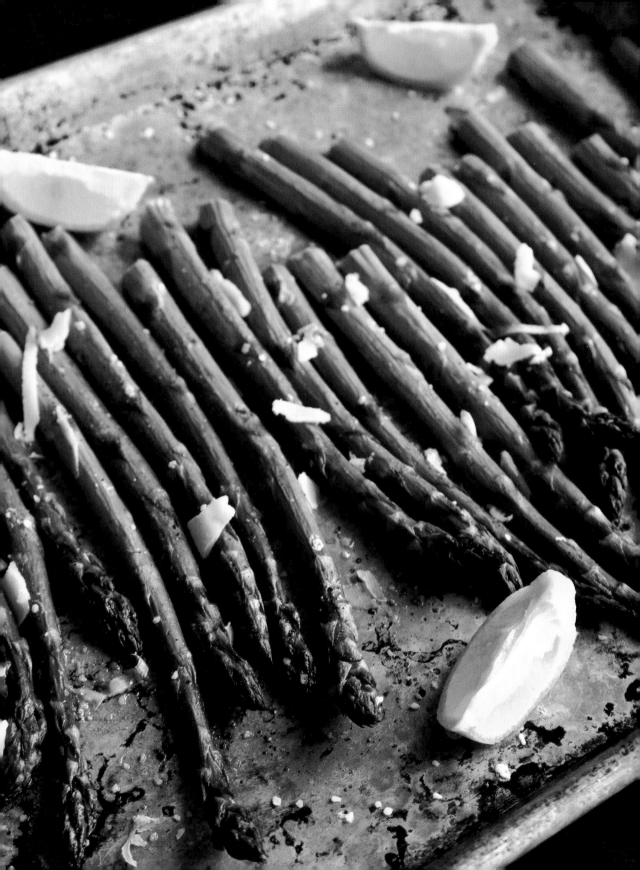

# Parmesan Roasted Asparagus

You can never go wrong serving roasted asparagus as a side dish. My favorite way to prepare it is by roasting it in the oven with a little bit of olive oil, salt, and pepper. But when I feel like getting a wee bit fancy, I'll sprinkle on some Parmesan cheese and top the asparagus with fresh-squeezed lemon juice for a tangy kick.

1. Preheat the oven to 450°F.

2. Place the asparagus in a single layer on a baking sheet. Drizzle the spears with the olive oil, and sprinkle with salt and pepper. Roast the asparagus for 10 minutes, or until tender but still crisp.

3. Arrange the spears on a serving platter, top them off with shaved Parmesan and a squeeze of lemon juice, and garnish with lemon wedges.

*Just for fun:* Substitute feta or blue cheese for the Parmesan.

**SERVES 4**

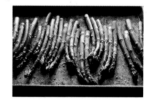

1 pound asparagus spears, trimmed

2 tablespoons extra-virgin olive oil

Kosher salt and freshly ground black pepper

Shaved Parmesan cheese, for garnish

½ lemon

Lemon wedges, for garnish

# Grilled Top Sirloin Steaks with Herbed Butter

When I was a kid my uncle would cook steaks until they were as tough as leather. Consequently, I believed that great-tasting, tender steaks were available only in upscale restaurants. It wasn't until I married my husband that I learned that not only was it possible to cook flavorful, juicy steaks at home, it was actually very easy. Now my favorite way to serve steak is with a generous pat of herbed garlic butter. This special touch will make you feel as if you're at a restaurant without even leaving your home!

**SERVES 4**

### STEAK

**4 teaspoons kosher salt**

**1 teaspoon freshly ground black pepper**

**½ teaspoon dried oregano**

**Grated zest from 1 lemon**

**Extra-virgin olive oil**

**Four 4-ounce boneless top sirloin steaks**

### HERBED BUTTER

**8 tablespoons (1 stick) unsalted butter, at room temperature**

**3 garlic cloves, minced**

**2 tablespoons minced fresh parsley**

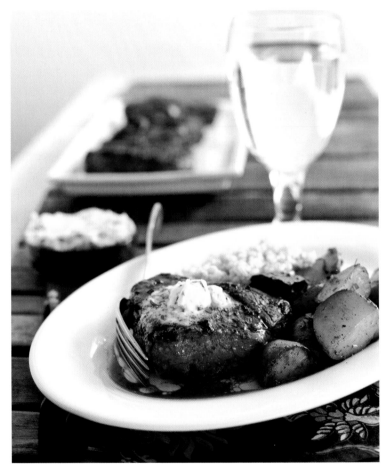

1.  In a small bowl, combine the salt, pepper, oregano, and lemon zest. Rub the seasonings between your thumb and index finger to infuse the salt with the oils from the lemon zest. Brush both sides of the steaks with olive oil. Then rub the spice blend on each side of the steaks and set aside.

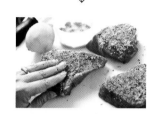

2.  Heat a gas grill or grill pan on high heat.

3.  While the grill is heating, prepare the herbed butter: Combine the butter, garlic, and parsley in a small bowl, blending thoroughly. Transfer the herbed butter to a small container and refrigerate until you're ready to use it.

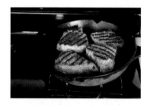

4.  Using tongs, carefully oil the grill with a paper towel soaked with olive oil. Place the steaks on the grill and cook for 5 to 6 minutes on each side for medium-rare. (If you prefer to use an internal meat thermometer, the ideal temperature is 130°F.) Remove the steaks, place them on a plate, and cover them loosely with aluminum foil. Allow the steaks to rest for 5 minutes.

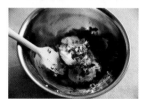

5.  Place each steak on a serving plate, and spoon some juices on top. Place a dollop of herbed butter on each steak before serving.

*Leftovers?* Chop leftover steak and use it in soups, fried rice, or omelets, or slice it for a sandwich. Use leftover herbed butter on hot rustic bread with any meal.

# Nutella Molten Lava Cakes

Hey, chocolate-lovers, meet your new best friend! These little molten lava cakes are warm, gooey, and filled with Nutella goodness. I always look forward to cracking open one of these little cakes with my fork and watching all the chocolate lava sauce ooze out. I love how each bite melts in my mouth, satisfying my chocolate craving and my sweet tooth simultaneously.

**SERVES 12**

### CAKES

**10 tablespoons (1¼ sticks) unsalted butter**

**1 cup semisweet chocolate chips**

**⅓ cup Nutella (chocolate-hazelnut spread)**

**½ cup all-purpose flour**

**1¼ cups confectioners' sugar**

**3 large eggs**

**3 egg yolks**

**1 teaspoon pure vanilla extract**

### GARNISH

**2 tablespoons confectioners' sugar**

**Nutella**

**Sweetened whipped cream (optional)**

**12 whole hazelnuts, toasted**

**6 fresh strawberries, sliced in half**

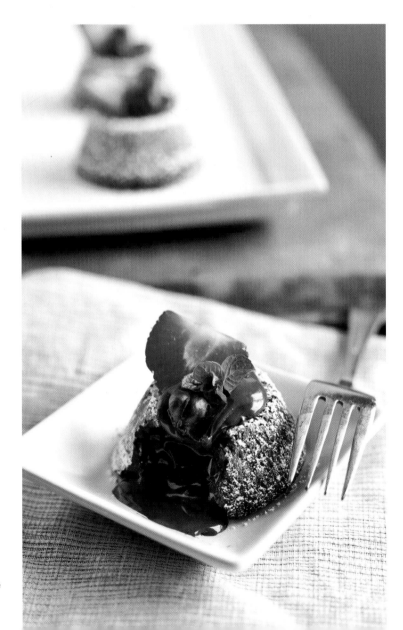

1. Preheat the oven to 375°F. Generously spray a 12-cup muffin tin with nonstick cooking spray.

2. Place the butter, chocolate chips, and Nutella in a large microwave-safe bowl. Heat the mixture in the microwave for 60 seconds, and then in three 30-second increments, stirring it until smooth after each interval. Stir the flour and confectioners' sugar into the chocolate-butter mixture. Mix in the eggs and egg yolks, one at a time. Add the vanilla and mix until combined.

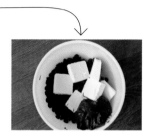

3. Divide the batter evenly among the muffin cups, filling them about three-quarters full. Bake for 8 to 10 minutes, or until the edges are firm but the centers are still soft.

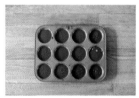

4. Allow the cakes to cool in the pan for 3 minutes to set up. Run a knife around the edges to loosen the cakes, and invert them onto a cutting board. Transfer each cake to a serving plate. Lightly dust confectioners' sugar over each one, followed by a dollop of Nutella, some sweetened whipped cream, if desired, a hazelnut, and a strawberry half.

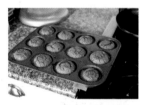

*Make ahead:* Molten lava batter can be made up to a week in advance. Spoon the batter into the muffin tin and cover it with plastic wrap. Store it in the refrigerator until you're ready to bake them. Set the muffin tin on the counter while the oven is preheating. The baking time will be the same.

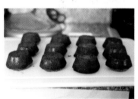

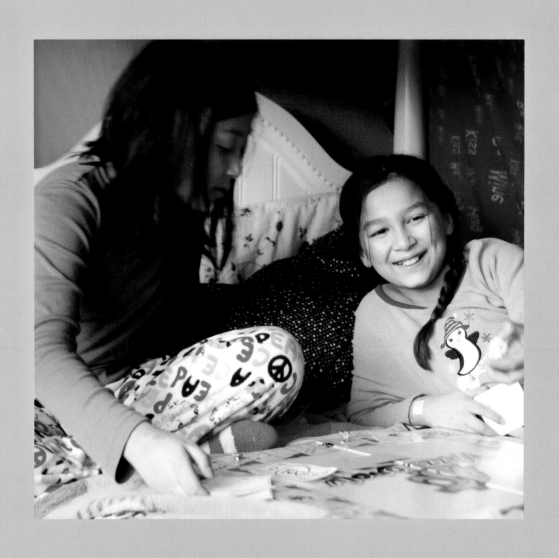

# eighteen

# FAMILY GAME NIGHT

We take family game night seriously around our house. Whether we're play-ing classic board games like Monopoly, Life, or mancala, or find ourselves in a dance-off on the Wii, one thing is for sure: bragging rights are on the line. No one wants to be on the receiving end of nightlong renditions of "We Are the Champions."

Long gone are the days when Rob and I would let Abbi and Mimi win as we tried to demonstrate what it looks like to win and lose graciously. The girls are now old enough to do some serious trash talking, with the skills to back it up. Make no mistake, they're fierce competitors and they know it! But they're also gracious when they lose . . . that is, if you call ignoring the winners' boastful chants gracious.

We love starting our game-filled evening with a fun Latin-inspired meal. I usually make a double batch of everything just in case friends stop by at the last minute, though these meals also work great as leftovers. After all, who wants to be cooking the next day when I have a Galaga title I must defend from my husband? Oh yes, I am the Galaga Queen—no one in my family (yes, Rob, I'm talking to you!) can beat me. And you wonder where my girls get their competitive spirit!

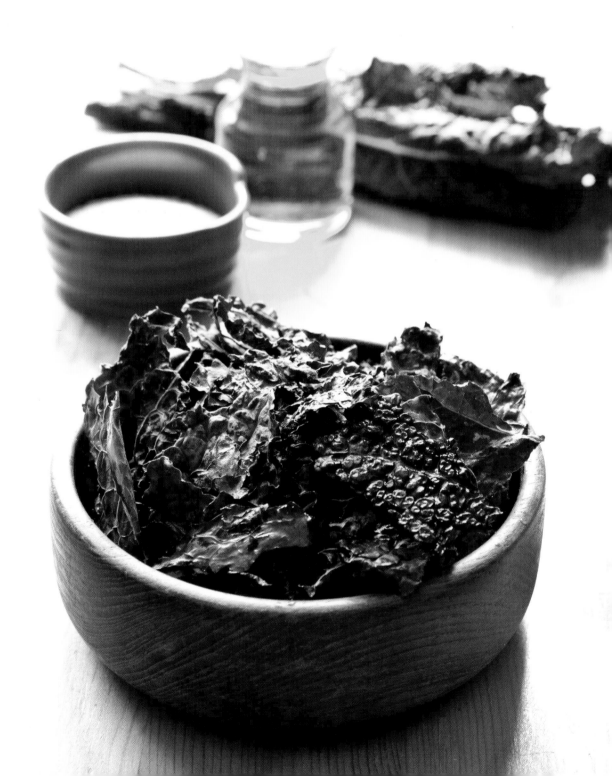

# Baked Kale Chips

Believe it or not, kale can be used to make crispy chips that the whole family will love. My kids were particularly skeptical the first time I tried serving them a batch, but now they love them almost as much as potato chips. It's one of those snack foods you can feel good about serving to your family.

1. Preheat the oven to 400°F. Line a baking sheet with parchment paper.

2. Tear the leafy part of the kale away from its rib and cut into bite-size pieces. Rinse it well and dry in a salad spinner. Discard the ribs. Transfer the kale to a mixing bowl and toss it with the olive oil.

3. Spread the kale in a single layer on the baking sheet. Season it lightly with salt. Bake for 15 minutes, or until crispy.

*Just for fun:* For a spicy twist, add 2 teaspoons balsamic vinegar and a touch of cayenne pepper when tossing with the olive oil.

**MAKES 2 TO 4 SERVINGS**

**1 bunch kale**
**2 tablespoons extra-virgin olive oil**
**Kosher salt**

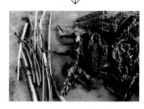

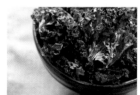

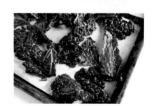

# Red Cabbage Pico de Gallo Salad

What do you get when you combine coleslaw and fresh pico de gallo? One fantastic side dish that adds a spicy kick to any meal. This vibrant salad is not only beautiful—it's healthy, too!

**SERVES 6 TO 8**

¼ cup extra-virgin olive oil

Juice from 3 limes

4 garlic cloves, minced

1 medium red cabbage, shredded

1 onion, chopped

2 cups cherry or grape tomatoes, halved

2 jalapeño peppers, seeded and minced

1 cup chopped fresh cilantro

1. To make the dressing, blend the olive oil, lime juice, and garlic in a mini food processor or blender, and set aside.

2. In a large bowl, combine the cabbage, onion, tomatoes, jalapeños, and cilantro. Pour the dressing over the salad ingredients and gently toss everything together. Allow the salad to absorb the dressing for 5 minutes before serving.

*Time-saving tip:* Shredded green cabbage, already washed and packed, can be found in the produce section of the grocery store. Although it isn't as vibrant as the red cabbage, it still makes a great salad!

*Just for fun:* To make great fish tacos, fill each taco with a small amount of this salad, a piece of grilled whitefish, and a little bit of tartar sauce. Or try the salad in Slow-Cooker Pulled Pork Tacos (page 258).

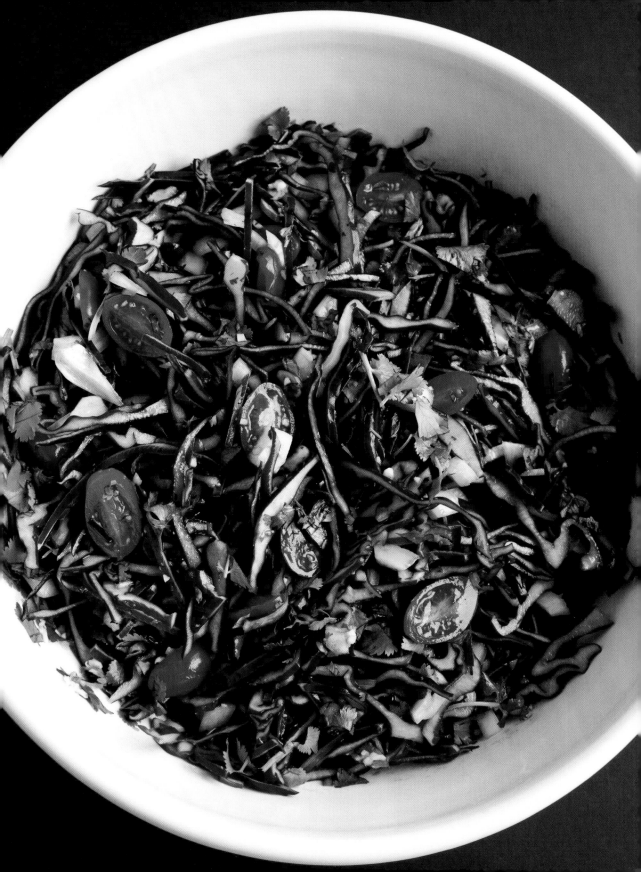

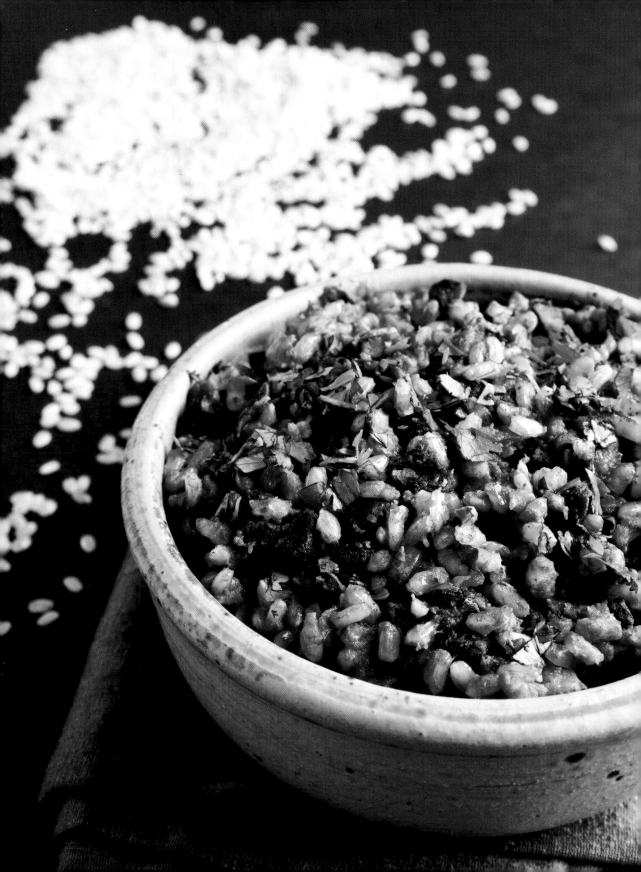

# Black Beans and Brown Rice

This recipe was inspired by my daughter Mimi, who decided one night to mix the black beans on her plate with the side of brown rice we were serving. By combining both dishes, we discovered how much more flavorful the two were when married together. Since then, I've loved making this dish. It's one of my favorite comfort food discoveries—and I owe it all to Mimi.

**SERVES 6 TO 8**

1. Add 2 tablespoons of the olive oil to a large heavy-duty pot set over medium heat. Add the onion, garlic, and salt, and sauté for 5 minutes, or until the onion has softened. Stir in the cumin, coriander, oregano, and chili powder. Add the remaining 2 tablespoons olive oil and the brown rice, and cook for 3 minutes, or until the rice is a bit softened. Increase the heat to medium-high and add the black beans, 2¼ cups water, and the bouillon cubes. Cover the pot, bring to a boil, and cook for 5 minutes.

2. Reduce the heat to a low simmer and cook for 50 to 60 minutes, until the rice is tender, stirring halfway through the cooking time. Fluff the rice and beans with a fork before serving.

*Cook's note:* If you have a large rice cooker, follow the recipe instructions through cooking the rice in the oil. Then transfer the rice and all the other ingredients to the rice cooker to finish cooking.

*Got leftovers?* A plate of rice and beans topped with a fried egg and served with a side of salsa makes a great breakfast.

**Ingredients:**

- 4 tablespoons extra-virgin olive oil
- 1 medium onion, finely chopped
- 4 garlic cloves, minced
- ½ teaspoon kosher salt
- 1½ tablespoons ground cumin
- ½ tablespoon ground coriander
- 2 teaspoons dried oregano
- 1 teaspoon chili powder
- 1½ cups uncooked brown rice
- Two 14-ounce cans black beans, rinsed and drained
- 2 chicken-flavored bouillon cubes

# Slow-Cooker Pulled Pork Tacos

I love using my slow cooker for braising meat without fuss—you just marinate the meat the night before and then toss everything into the slow cooker the next morning before you leave for work. By the time you come home, dinner is ready—and the house smells incredible. Pulled pork can be used for many dishes, but one of my favorite ways to eat it is as a taco filling in warm soft corn tortillas with a side of rice and beans. It's so nice to let the slow cooker do all the work—and what a mighty fine job it does!

**SERVES 6 TO 8**

3 pounds boneless pork shoulder, cut into 3-inch chunks

3 tablespoons dark brown sugar

1 tablespoon ground cumin

1 tablespoon ground coriander

2 teaspoons garlic salt

2 teaspoons smoked paprika

1 teaspoon dried oregano

½ cup soy sauce

¼ cup distilled white vinegar

1 medium onion, chopped

1 package corn tortillas (24 count)

1. Place the pork in a medium bowl. In a separate bowl, combine the brown sugar, cumin, coriander, garlic salt, smoked paprika, and oregano to make a rub. Add the spice mixture to the pork and massage it into the meat with your hands until the dry mix adheres to the pork. Place the pork in a large plastic freezer bag, and add the soy sauce and vinegar. Set the pork in the refrigerator to marinate overnight.

2. Scatter the onions over the bottom of the slow cooker, and then add the pork and marinade. Cook on low heat for 8 to 10 hours, until the meat shreds easily.

3. Remove the meat from the slow cooker and pull it apart with two forks. Baste the shredded meat with the liquid remaining in the slow cooker to keep it moist. Spoon the shredded pork into the corn tortillas, add your choice of fixins (see below), and devour!

*Taco fixins:* Enjoy the pulled pork tacos with fresh guacamole, pico de gallo, shredded Monterey Jack cheese, cilantro, fresh lime juice, sliced radishes, shredded lettuce, chopped tomatoes, and/or salsa.

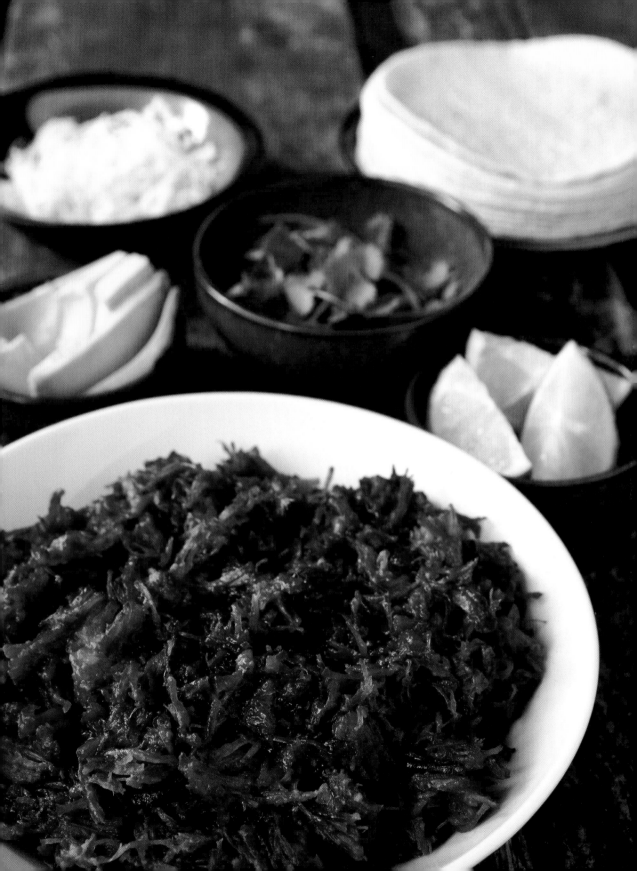

# The Best Chocolate Chip Cookies Ever

It's a bold claim to publicly declare my chocolate chip cookies to be the best ever. Just know that I wouldn't say this if I didn't really believe it. And many other people believe it too, because this has become one of the most popular chocolate chip cookie recipes on the Internet! What makes them so special? They aren't too sweet, have crispy bottoms and soft, chewy centers, and are loaded with chocolate chips and a hint of sea salt in every bite. These cookies are truly magnificent.

**MAKES 4 DOZEN COOKIES**

1 cup (2 sticks) unsalted butter, at room temperature

½ cup granulated sugar

1½ cups firmly packed dark brown sugar

2 eggs

2 teaspoons pure vanilla extract

2¾ cups all-purpose flour

1½ teaspoons baking powder

1 teaspoon baking soda

¾ teaspoon sea salt

2¼ cups semisweet chocolate chips

1. Preheat the oven to 360°F. Line a cookie sheet with parchment paper.

2. Using a hand or stand mixer, cream the butter, granulated sugar, and brown sugar together on medium-high speed for 3 minutes, until nice and fluffy. Beat in the eggs one at a time, then add the vanilla, and mix for 2 minutes. Reduce the mixer speed to medium-low and add the flour, baking powder, baking soda, and salt. When the cookie dough has absorbed the dry ingredients, stir in the chocolate chips and mix until they are well distributed.

3. Drop 2 tablespoons of dough (or use a medium cookie scoop) onto the cookie sheet for each cookie, spacing them 2 inches apart. Bake for 15 minutes, or until the edges are nice and golden brown. Remove the cookie sheet from the oven and allow the cookies to cool for 2 minutes. Then slide the parchment paper, with the cookies still on top, onto a wire rack to cool completely.

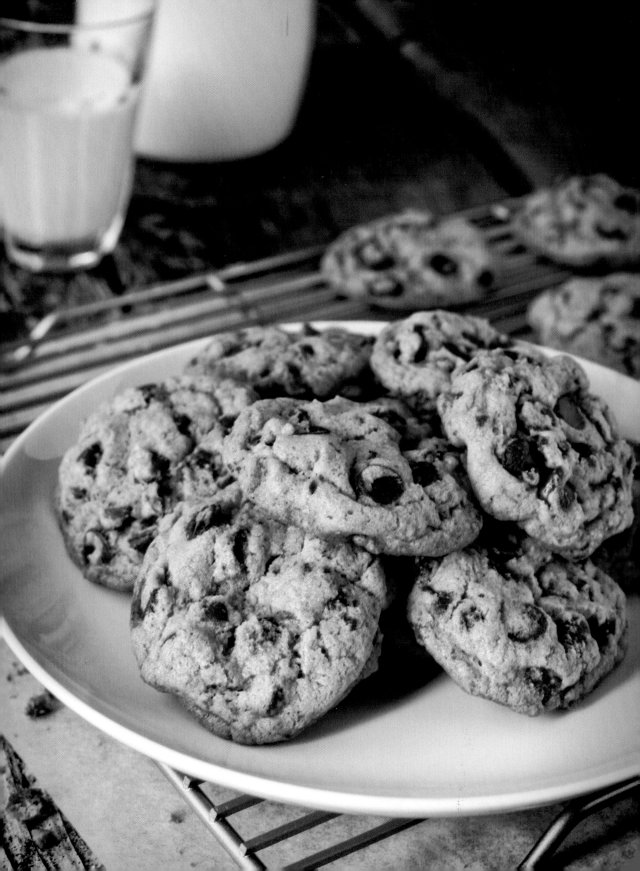

*Cook's note:* Kosher salt can be substituted for the sea salt.

*Why 360°F?* The loss of heat when the oven door opens affects the rise of the cookie dough. By increasing the oven temperature, the cookies bake slightly higher and develop a nice crispy edge while the inside remains soft.

*Just for fun:* Add 1 cup chopped nuts for added crunch and flavor. I love using walnuts, almonds, pecans, or macadamia nuts.

*Troubleshooting:* If your cookies turn out flat, here are some possible reasons:

- Your baking powder and/or baking soda is old and expired. If either of these ingredients is more than a year old and has not been stored in a sealed (preferably airtight) container, it has likely lost its leavening power.

- It's not enough to just cream the butter and sugars until they have come together. This recipe requires you to mix them for at least 3 minutes, until the texture is light and fluffy.

# ACKNOWLEDGMENTS

*I was deeply* uplifted by all the people who surrounded me with their love, support, and encouragement while writing this cookbook—especially after my father's passing.

My wonderful husband, Rob, and my beloved children, Abbi, Mimi, and Eli, who fill my heart with abundant joy daily.

The fabulous readers of Savory Sweet Life, who have supported me from the very conception of the site. I love you guys and appreciate each and every one of you!

My talented literary agent, Meg Thompson, who is more like a friend than an agent. Her honesty, encouragement, enthusiasm, and advocacy for me every step of the way made it possible for me to set worries aside and be excited about everything.

My fantastic editor, Cassie Jones, for believing in a Savory Sweet Life cookbook. Her easygoing disposition and professional expertise allowed me to enjoy the process of writing and photographing this book. Collaborating with her was truly enjoyable, and her creative input was invaluable.

Assistant editor Jessica McGrady, who consistently helped me stay on task and worked on many behind-the-scenes details to produce a book I could be proud of, and the publishing team at William Morrow, including Liate Stehlik, Lynn Grady, Tavia Kowalchuk, Shawn Nicholls, Lorie Young, Lorie Pagnozzi, and Karen Lumley, who worked so diligently on this project.

Ree Drummond, who offered constant encouragement, words of wisdom, and heartfelt friendship.

My colleagues at PBS Parents, Tracey Wynne and Aviva Goldfarb, who are a pleasure to work with and a joy to share great food with every week on Kitchen Explorers.

Cathy Herholdt, who made it a priority to look over my manuscript before sending it off to my publisher. Thank you, Cathy!

My dear friends Allison, Michelle, Keren, Betsy, Emily, Jeni, Stacy, Lisa, Ashley, Rebekah, Pam, Maggy, Erika, Aran, Amanda, Jill, Sarah, Susie, Francine, Ginny, and the ladies in my Moms in Touch group, who are the very definition of friends who love at all times.

The Currah, Sorrell, Chew, Cook, Mark, O, Mayfield, Quraishi, Haven, Astion, Crum, Gallagher, Koontz, and Howland families, who have been a constant source of love and encouragement.

My siblings, Joyce, Bryan, Grace, Eunice, and Janice, with whom I have always shared much love, laughter, and great food.

Last and most important, my mom, for being the very definition of grace and humility. "Many women do noble things, but you surpass them all." —Proverbs 31:29

# RECIPES BY CATEGORY

Corn Pudding
Garlic Cheese Bread
Parmesan Roasted Asparagus
Roasted Carrots with Sage Brown
    Butter
Roasted Skillet Potatoes
Sautéed Swiss Chard
Scalloped Potato Leek Gratin
Stir-Fry Garlic Ginger Broccoli

### DESSERTS

All-Occasion Vanilla Cake with
    Buttercream Frosting and Sour
    Cream Raspberry Filling
Banana Cream Pie
The Best Chocolate Chip Cookies
    Ever

Blackberry Crisp
Chocolate Chocolate Chip Banana
    Bread
Chocolate Cookies 'n' Cream
    Dairy-Free "Ice Cream"
Chocolate Cupcakes with Peanut
    Butter Cookie Frosting
Dad's Carrot Cake
Daiquiri Lime Ice Pops
Heavenly Almond Pound Cake
Irresistible Ganache Brownies
Mango Frozen Yogurt Pops
Nutella Molten Lava Cakes
Nutella, Strawberry, and Banana
    Crêpes
Oven-Broiled S'mores
Pint-Size Biscotti

Pretty in Pink Marshmallow Pops
Rustic Spiced Plum Tart
Soft Chocolate Gingersnap
    Cookies

### BEVERAGES

Blueberry Oat Smoothie
Coffee Frappe
Eggnog Coffee
Old-Fashioned Root Beer Floats
Peaches 'n' Cream Italian Cream
    Soda
Rich Hot Chocolate
Sparkling Cranberry Rum Punch
Strawberry Lemonade
Thai Iced Tea

# INDEX

641.5
CUR
Currah, Alice.

Savory sweet life.

AUG 1 4 2012